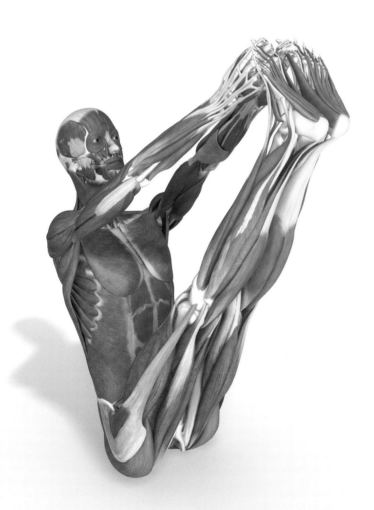

"On a given day, a given circumstance, you think you have a limit. And you then go for this limit and you touch this limit, and you think, 'Okay, this is the limit.' As soon as you touch this limit, something happens and you suddenly can go a little bit further. With your mind power, your determination, your instinct, and the experience as well, you can fly very high."

– Ayrton Senna

Written by Raymond A. Long, MD, FRCSC; Illustrated by Chris Macivor

Design: Chris Cantley

Ten Bull Pictures Illustrated by Alana McCarthy

Editorial Services: Anne McDonell, Eileen Wolfberg

Proofreader: Eryn Kirkwood, MA

Copyright ©2008, Raymond A Long, MD, FRCSC

ISBN 13: 978-1-60743-239-5

Bandha Yoga Publications

About the Author

Ray Long, MD, FRCSC, is a board certified orthopedic surgeon and the author of "The Key Muscles of Hatha Yoga." Ray graduated from The University of Michigan Medical School with post-graduate training at Cornell University, McGill University, The University of Montreal, and Florida Orthopedic Institute. Ray has studied Hatha Yoga for over 20 years, travelling to India on numerous occasions to study extensively with B.K.S. Iyengar and other leading Yoga masters.

About the Illustrator

Chris Macivor has been involved in the field of digital content creation for well over 10 years. He is a graduate of Etobicoke School of the Arts, Sheridan College, and Seneca College. Chris considers himself to be equally artistic and technical in nature. As such, his work has spanned many genres from film and television to videogames and underwater imagery. Working with Dr. Long on the "Scientific Keys" book series, he has endeavored to digitally reproduce the biomechanical perfection of the human body. With a keen eye for subtle lighting and a passion to strive for excellence in his art, Chris constantly seeks to bring his imagery to life.

Table of Contents

Introduction

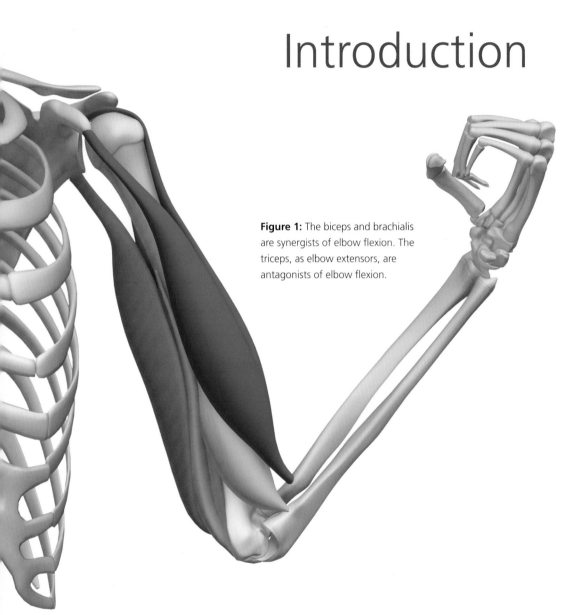

Figure 1: The biceps and brachialis are synergists of elbow flexion. The triceps, as elbow extensors, are antagonists of elbow flexion.

My first spiritual teacher, author and mystic Robert A. Johnson, taught me to "look at what is." He was speaking about life in general, and his advice applies to the practice of Hatha Yoga as well.

Throughout our first book in this series, "The Key Muscles of Hatha Yoga," we illustrate the relationship between form and function for the bones, joints, ligaments, and muscles. Similarly, looking at the form or shape of any given Yoga pose reveals its unique function.

Individual joints have a number of specific muscles that create movement. Look at Figure 1 to see how activating the biceps and brachialis muscles flexes the elbow and lengthens the muscles that oppose this action—those at the back of the upper arm, the triceps.

Individual Yoga poses have specific groups of muscles that work together to create optimal form. I call these muscle groups the synergists of the pose. You can deepen and stabilize a pose by activating these muscles.

Look at Figure 2 to see this concept in action with the standing pose Prasarita Padottanasana. This image illustrates how contracting the muscles at the front of the thigh, hip, and torso—the quadriceps, psoas, and rectus abdominis—deepens the pose and stretches the opposing muscles at the back of the thigh and buttocks and along the spine. This is how combining the synergists in a Yoga pose creates the optimal functional benefit for the practitioner.

Yoga poses are like "keys" that unlock our conscious awareness of the body. Forward bends stretch and release the structures on the back of the body, while strengthening the muscles on the front of the body. Back bends have an opposite effect, and so on for the different categories of poses. Knowledge of the functional anatomy of Yoga reveals the mechanisms behind these processes.

"The Key Poses of Hatha Yoga" is intended to be a visual reference for the practitioner to aid in his or her individual journey. It illustrates 55 of the fundamental poses of Hatha Yoga, the suggested positions of the major joints and muscles that contract to create these key positions, as well as the muscles that stretch in the various poses. Part One of "The Key Poses of Hatha Yoga" illustrates the science behind the biomechanics and physiology of stretching muscles. Part Two applies this knowledge to the various categories of poses to unlock the benefits.

Practicing Yoga is an exploration of our individual bodies. Bear in mind that there are many interpretations of the poses. There are also variations for the postures, depending on the system of Hatha Yoga and the experience of the practitioner. Enjoy your practice and seek out your own "best" interpretations. Find out what works for you in opening the door to your individual experience of Yoga.

Namasté

Ray Long, MD, FRCSC

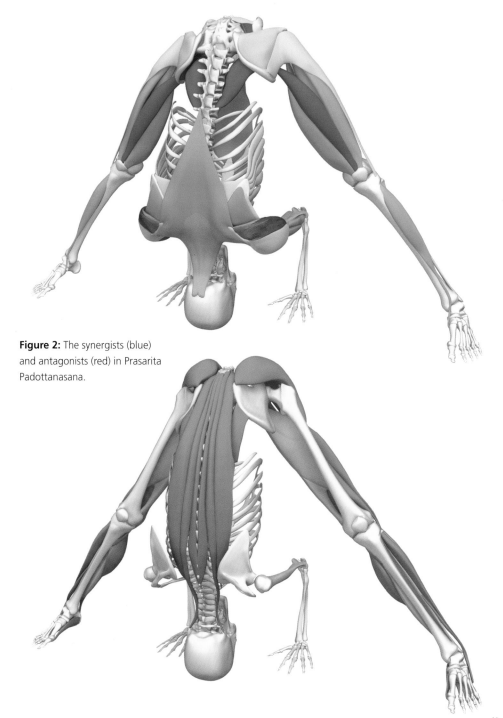

Figure 2: The synergists (blue) and antagonists (red) in Prasarita Padottanasana.

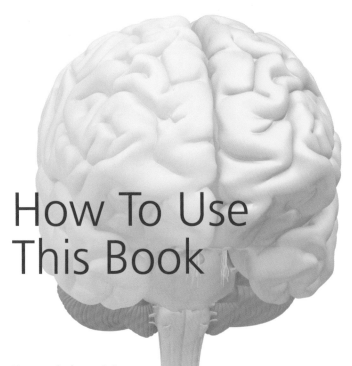

How To Use This Book

Practicing Yoga using the right side of the brain

Visual artists often approach their subjects using the right side of their brain. This is because the right brain is concerned with creativity and spatial awareness. When an artist undertakes to draw an elbow, for example, he or she will often discard preconceived ideas of how an elbow should look and switch to a visual mode of thought. Artists do this by thinking in terms of forms, angles, light, and shadow. What emerges is a unique image. This concept is well described by author Dr. Betty Edwards in her groundbreaking work "Drawing on the Right Side of the Brain."

Practicing Yoga can be approached in much the same way. For example, looking at the form of Downward Dog Pose reveals that the arms and legs are straight and the hips are flexed. We can make our own rendition of this pose by activating the muscles that best create this form. In this case, we contract the triceps to straighten the elbows, the quadriceps to straighten the knees, and the hip flexors to bend the torso. This process can be applied to any Yoga pose through a basic knowledge of functional anatomy. In this way, we can use the musculoskeletal system to create the forms of Yoga with the body, much as one would use a brush or chisel to create a work of art. This results in a cognitive shift to visual right brain thinking and evokes a trance-like meditative state.

"The Key Poses of Hatha Yoga" illustrates a variety of the suggested muscles that can be activated or relaxed to deepen and improve Yoga poses. First take a "Gestalt" approach and simply enjoy the images, allowing them to permeate your unconscious mind. Then begin to break the poses down by looking at specific joints and experimenting with the muscles surrounding them.

The Sanskrit word for focus is "Drishti." Use your knowledge of the body to create Drishti in your practice. I recommend limiting your concentration to one muscle group at a time in any given pose. Focus on the large muscles at first to create a specific movement, and then use the smaller muscles to refine the movement. Go slowly and gently, consolidating your knowledge of anatomy and physiology over time. Remember that your brain will unconsciously integrate what you learn during the time between your practices.

Above all, have fun and practice safely.

Part One: Theory

Use Part One to learn about the science behind the biomechanics and physiology of Yoga.

Part Two: Practice

Use Part Two to learn about the specific poses. Muscles that are activating (contracting) are colored blue, and muscles that are stretching are red. Most poses also have an inset image detailing some aspect of the musculoskeletal system in that particular pose.

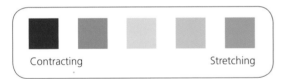

Contracting   Stretching

Appendix A:
Guide to Body Movement

Use Appendix A as a reference for individual joint movement.

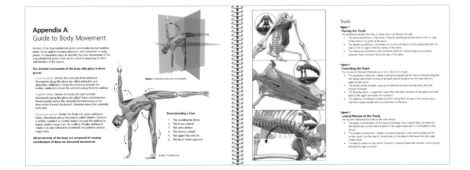

Appendix B:
Index of Anatomy

Use Appendix B to review muscle and bone names and locations on the body. For more detailed information on musculoskeletal anatomy in relation to Yoga, Volume I of this series, "The Key Muscles of Hatha Yoga," is recommended.

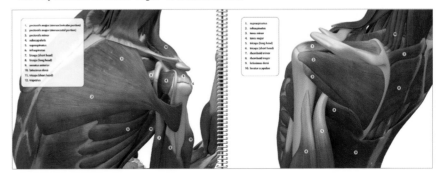

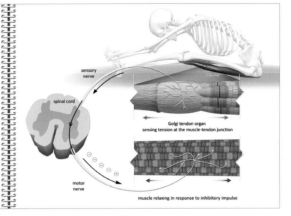

Golgi Tendon Organ

The Golgi tendon organ is a sensory receptor or motion detector that is located where the muscle and tendon are joined. It detects changes in tension, and when tension increases, signals the muscle to relax. This acts like a "circuit breaker" to prevent injury to the tendon when tension generated by the contracting muscle becomes too high. This contrasts with the muscle spindle receptor, which detects change in length and signals the muscle to contract.

The Golgi tendon organ forms the basis for a phenomenon used by physical therapists and sports trainers known as proprioceptive neuromuscular facilitation or "PNF". In PNF we temporarily contract a target muscle that we are trying to stretch in order to stimulate the Golgi tendon organ. The Golgi tendon organ then signals the muscle to relax. In effect, this creates "slack" in the muscle that we can then take up by going deeper into the stretch.

This may seem counterintuitive at first–contracting a muscle that we are trying to stretch; however, when applied carefully this technique can be used to "dissolve" blocks and deepen poses. To understand the technique, we will look at lengthening the hamstrings, the muscles down the back of the thigh in Janu Sirsasana. The technique is generally applied as follows:

1. First, take the muscle out to length. This establishes where the "set length" of the muscle is, the point that the brain recognizes as the end of the stretch.

2. Next, gently contract the target muscle. In this case, we are focusing on the hamstrings of the straight leg, so we attempt to bend the knee to create a contraction in the hamstrings (the action of the hamstrings is to bend the knee). I generally access this by slightly bending the knee and pressing the heel into the floor. This causes the hamstrings to contract.

3. Contract the muscle to no more than twenty percent of its maximum force and hold this for eight to ten seconds. Then relax for one breath.

4. Now, contract the antagonist muscles at the front of the thigh to take the target muscle out to a new length. In this case, we contract the quadriceps to straighten the knee and bend deeper into the stretch of the hamstrings.

Hints and cautions:

1. If you are new to yoga, spend a few months conditioning your body first before using these powerful techniques to deepen stretches.

2. Remember that the Golgi tendon organ is there to protect the tendon from injury, but its ability to protect the tendon has limits. Never overdo it when using this technique. Never contract the target muscle more than about twenty percent of its maximum force.

3. The force generated by contracting muscles is transmitted to the joints. This is called the "joint reaction force" so you must always protect your joints by maintaining them in their natural alignment while stretching. If you experience joint pain, then back off from the stretch and stop.

4. Focus on one muscle group at a time and limit your "PNF" stretching to one pose in a practice session. Do no more than two to three cycles of the stretch described above.

5. Allow ample time (forty eight hours) for recovery before repeating this technique.

6. Always practice under the guidance of an experienced and qualified teacher.

sensory nerve

spinal cord

Golgi tendon organ sensing tension at the muscle-tendon junction

motor nerve

muscle relaxing in response to inhibitory impulse

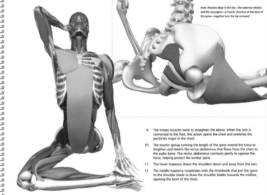

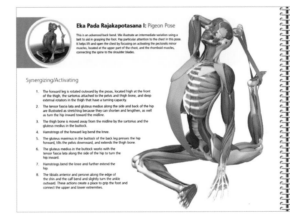

Eka Pada Rajakapotasana I: Pigeon Pose

This is an advanced back bend. We illustrate an intermediate variation using a belt to aid in grasping the foot. Pay particular attention to the chest in this pose. It helps lift and open the chest by focusing on activating the pectoralis minor muscles, located at the upper part of the chest, and the rhomboid muscles, connecting the spine to the shoulder blades.

Synergizing/Activating

1. The forward leg is rotated outward by the psoas, located high at the front of the thigh, the sartorius attached to the pelvis and thigh bone, and deep external rotators in the thigh that have a turning capacity.

2. The tensor fascia lata and gluteus medius along the side and back of the hip are illustrated as stretching because they can shorten and lengthen, as well as turn the hip inward toward the midline.

3. The thigh bone is moved away from the midline by the sartorius and the gluteus medius in the buttock.

4. Hamstrings of the forward leg bend the knee.

5. The gluteus maximus in the buttock of the back leg presses the hip forward, tilts the pelvis downward, and extends the thigh bone.

6. The gluteus medius in the buttock works with the tensor fascia lata along the side of the hip to turn the hip inward.

7. Hamstrings bend the knee and further extend the hip.

8. The tibialis anterior and peroneus along the edge of the shin and the calf bend and slightly turn the ankle outward. These actions create a place to grip the foot and connect the upper and lower extremities.

9. The triceps muscles work to straighten the elbow. When the arm is connected to the foot, this action opens the chest and stretches the pectoralis major in the chest.

10. The erector spinae running the length of the spine extend the torso to lengthen and stretch the rectus abdominus that flows from the chest to the pubic bone. The rectus abdominus contracts gently to oppose this force, helping protect the lumbar spine.

11. The lower trapezius draws the shoulders down and away from the ears.

12. The middle trapezius cooperates with the rhomboids that join the spine to the shoulder blade to draw the shoulder blades towards the midline, opening the front of the chest.

Insert: Muscles deep in the hip—the external rotation and the coccygeus—a muscle structure at the base of the spine—together turn the hip outward.

Part One: Theory

Biomechanics of Stretching

A number of years ago, I asked the great Yoga master, B.KS. Iyengar, what he thought was the key to mastering Yoga. In response, he held up one hand and, pointing to each of the different surfaces of his fingers, the insides, the outsides, front and back, said: "You must balance all of the energies in each part of the body."

The Sanskrit word "Hatha" means Sun/Moon and implies a balanced Yin/Yang in Yoga. Viewed in this way, Mr. Iyengar's statement captures the essence of Hatha Yoga.

Understanding biomechanical processes and interactions is one key to balancing the forces and energies throughout the body. Body biomechanics are under the mind's conscious control. The brain controls the skeletal muscles that move the bones and joints, signaling the muscles to contract or relax and moving the body into the positions of Yoga.

Each joint is surrounded by muscles that are grouped according to the movement they produce when contracting or relaxing. The agonist or prime mover muscles act to produce a given movement. Synergist muscles aid with this movement, and antagonist muscles oppose it (Figure 1). Working in concert, these various muscles balance the energies in each part of the body.

Joint Mobility and Stability–The Biomechanical Yin/Yang

Joint mobility and stability function in a Yin/Yang fashion. The greater the mobility, the lesser the stability (and vice versa). Musculoskeletal biomechanics describe this process. Three factors determine movement about a given joint:

1. The bone shape
2. The capsuloligamentous structures
3. The muscles that surround the joint

The shape of the bones forming a joint contributes to determining its range of motion. A deep ball and socket joint, such as the hip, has limited movement in three planes and the stability to bear the body weight. A shallower ball and socket joint such as the shoulder has greater mobility than the hip, but far less stability (Figure 2).

The capsule and ligaments surrounding the joints are known as the capsuloligamentous structures. The joint capsule and ligaments are comprised of fibrous connective tissue. Capsuloligamentous structures fasten bones to one another and also contribute to determining joint mobility and stability. They function like mobile extensions of bones at the joint. Like the bones, the form of the capsuloligamentous structures reflects their function.

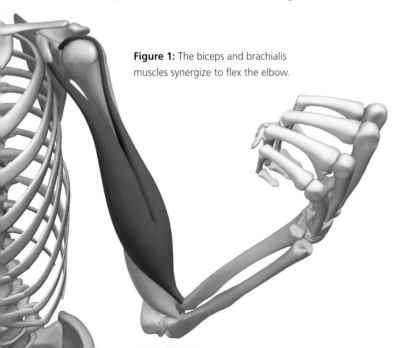

Figure 1: The biceps and brachialis muscles synergize to flex the elbow.

Bones forming stable joints, such as the sacroiliac joint, are held together by thick stout ligaments, allowing only limited joint mobility. On the other hand, bones forming the shoulder joint are connected by much thinner, more malleable ligaments, allowing greater mobility.

Finally, there are muscles that surround the joint—the muscular stabilizers. Contracting muscles not only produces movement but also stabilizes the joints. The contractile state of a muscle affects the mobility of the joint. Tight muscles limit joint mobility, and relaxed muscles increase it. Stretching lengthens the muscular stabilizers of a specific joint, allowing for greater range of motion of that joint. Practicing Yoga lengthens muscles surrounding multiple joints and increases the range of motion for the entire body.

Limitations in the ability to perform a given Yoga pose can result from any of the factors determining joint mobility and stability, including the muscle's contractile state, the length and/or tightness of the capsuloligamentous structures, and the bone shape—or a combination of these factors.

Bone shape is permanent and cannot be changed once the growth plates are closed (during adolescence). While the shapes of bones vary from person to person, it is difficult to say that a particular individual's bone shape is the limiting factor in their ability to perform a given Yoga pose. The state of the capsuloligamentous structures can also limit the ability to perform a Yoga pose. Furthermore, ligaments have a limited capacity to stretch without being damaged, potentially creating instability about the joint.

Since bone shape cannot be changed and ligament length should not be changed, we are left to work with the muscular stabilizers. This is a good thing. It simplifies matters because the length intention of skeletal muscles is under our conscious influence and can be safely affected by practicing Yoga to improve the body's range of motion.

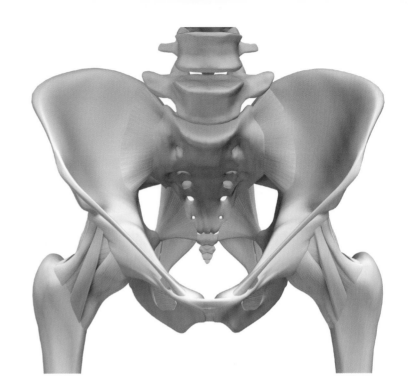

Figure 2: The deep ball and socket joint of the hip and the shallow ball and socket joint of the more mobile shoulder (with ligaments).

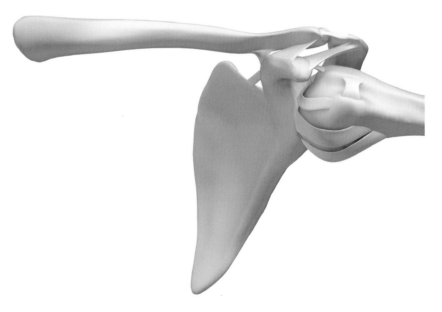

What is Stretching?

All skeletal muscles have an origin in one part of the skeleton and an insertion on another part. Stretching a muscle basically involves moving its origin and insertion farther apart. Muscles can be stretched by fixing their skeletal origin in place and moving the insertion, or vice versa (or a combination). The figures on these pages use the supraspinatus and hamstring muscles to illustrate this concept.

Here Garudasana (Eagle Pose) illustrates moving the origin or insertion of the supraspinatus muscle in the shoulder to create length.

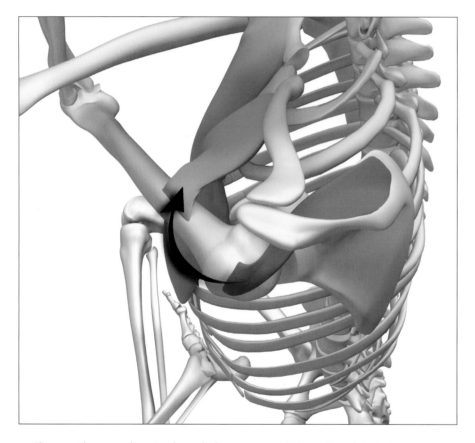 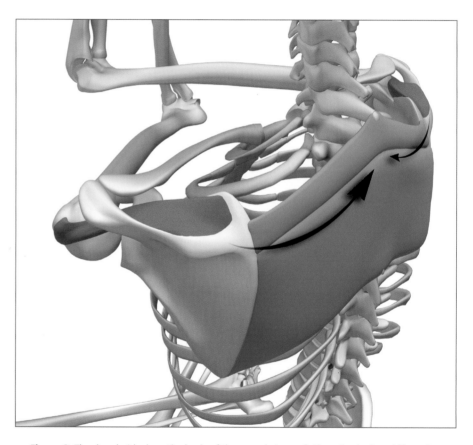

Figure 1: The pectoralis major draws the humerus towards the midline of the body. This action moves the insertion of the supraspinatus muscle on the head of the humerus away from its origin on the body of the scapula.

Figure 2: The rhomboids draw the body of the scapula towards the spine in the midline of the back. This action moves the origin of the supraspinatus muscle away from its insertion on the head of the humerus.

Several structures are affected when a muscle lengthens, including the connective tissue elements that ensheath the muscle and the contractile elements that cause it to contract. Connective tissues lengthen over time with consistent practice. The contractile elements (also known as myomeres) are under the control of the central nervous system. We focus on these elements in the section entitled "Physiology of Stretching."

Here Uttanasana illustrates moving the origin or insertion of the hamstrings to create length in the back of the thighs.

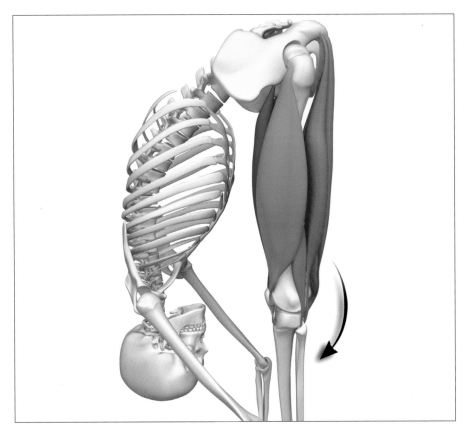

Figure 3: The quadriceps straighten the knees. This action moves the insertion of the hamstrings away from their origin on the ischial tuberosity of the pelvis.

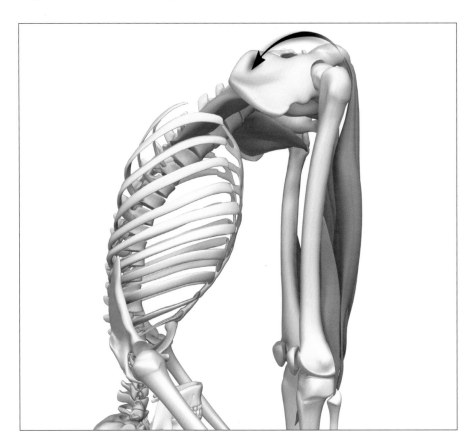

Figure 4: The psoas tilts the pelvis forward. This action draws the origin of the hamstring muscles at the back of the pelvis upwards and away from their insertion on the lower leg.

Moving Origins and Insertions

The following pages use Janu Sirsasana to illustrate moving the origins and insertions of a series of muscles throughout the body to deepen a pose.

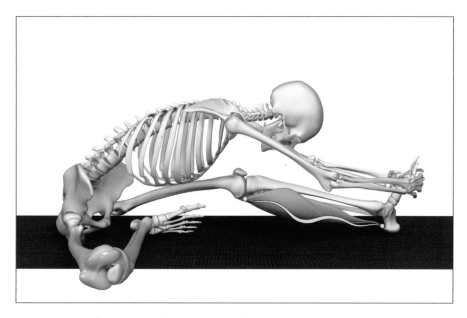

Figure 1: Bending the knee releases the origin of the main calf muscle, the gastrocnemius. This allows its insertion on the heel bone to move freely.

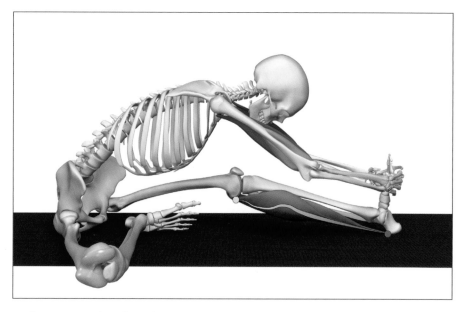

Figure 2: Once the calf muscles are relaxed, bend the elbows to tilt the foot backwards and hold it in this position. This fixes the insertion of the calf muscles at a point further away from their origin on the femur. This is an example of connecting the upper and lower extremities to deepen a pose.

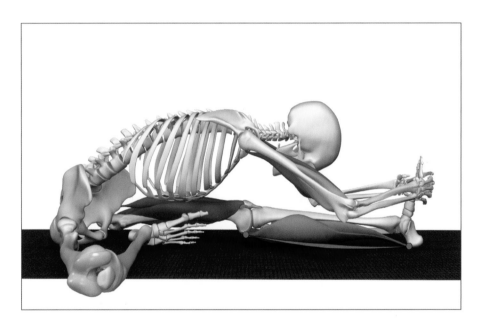

Figure 3: The hands continue to grip the feet while the biceps and brachialis muscles remain active, bending the elbows and holding the foot in the tilted back (dorsiflexed) position. The quadriceps then straighten the knee. This action draws the origin of the calf muscles on the back of the knee away from their insertion on the heel, stretching these muscles.

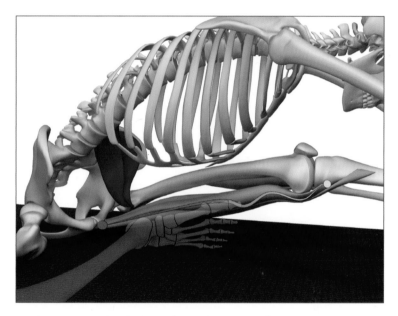

Figure 4-a: Bending the knee releases the insertion of the hamstring muscles on the lower leg. The psoas muscle then tilts the pelvis forward. This action moves the origin of the hamstrings at the back of the pelvis away from their insertion on the lower leg.

Moving Origins and Insertions

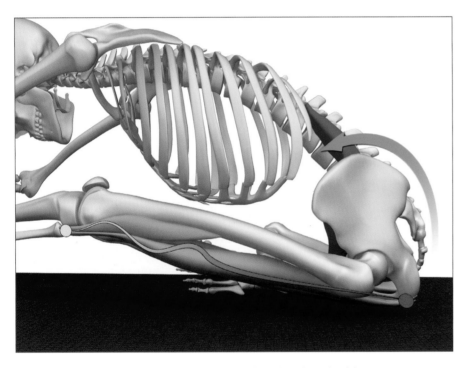

Figure 4-b: Here we show the same action as 4-a from the other side of the pose.

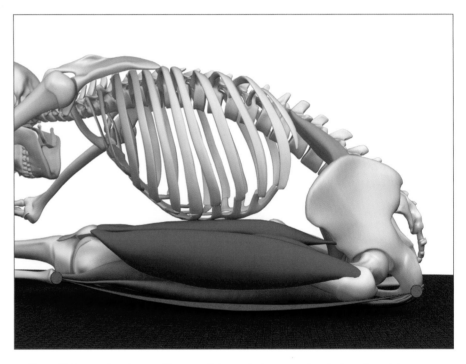

Figure 5: Contracting the quadriceps straightens the knee, moving the insertion of the hamstrings on the lower leg away from their origin at the back of the pelvis. The psoas maintains the pelvis in a tilted forward position. These actions combine to lengthen the hamstrings.

These images illustrate how Janu Sirsasana combines movements of the various major joints—the ankle, knee, hip, elbows, and those of the spine—to create length in the muscles of the back of the body.

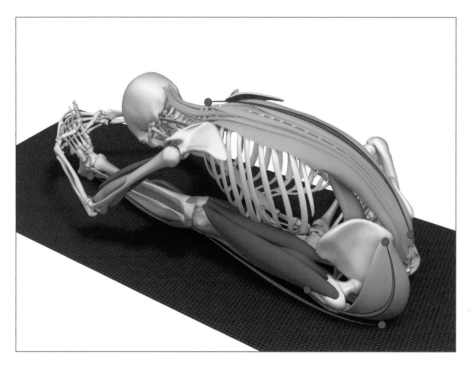
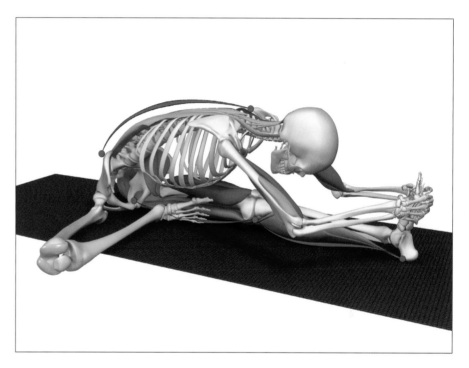

Figures 6-a, 6-b: The hands and arms tilt the ankle joint back and the knee straightens, lengthening the calf muscles. The knee straightens and the pelvis tilts forward, lengthening the hamstrings. The hip flexes, lengthening the gluteus maximus. The elbows flex, bending the trunk forward to stretch the muscles running the length of the spine. This action pulls the pelvis further forward and combines with the psoas to intensify the entire stretch.

Physiology of Stretching

Musculoskeletal biomechanics are under our conscious control. For example, when we want to straighten the knee, the brain signals the quadriceps to contract and the knee straightens, stretching the hamstrings. This action triggers a chain of physiological responses that take place without our conscious awareness.

Receptors within the joints and muscles detect movement and changes in muscle tension and length. These receptors signal the central nervous system, which responds by regulating the contractile state of the muscles. This, in turn, affects the range of motion of a given joint.

In this way, conscious biomechanical actions influence unconscious physiological responses. Moving the body into a Yoga posture initiates a cascade of these biomechanical and physiological events.

The Spinal Cord Reflexes

Spinal cord reflex arcs regulate the tension and length of skeletal muscle contractile elements. This regulation occurs automatically in response to biomechanical actions. When a muscle contracts or stretches, receptors within it alert the central nervous system to this event. The central nervous system then signals the muscle to respond appropriately, either by relaxing or by contracting. All of this takes place without our being aware of it by way of an arc of nerves between the muscles and the spinal cord. The result is a Yin/Yang feedback mechanism that balances and fine-tunes movement.

A complex array of receptors and their corresponding reflex arcs connect the musculoskeletal system to the central nervous system. For practical purposes, I have limited the discussion in this chapter to the three major spinal cord reflexes: the muscle spindle, reciprocal inhibition, and the Golgi tendon organ.

Methods of Stretching Muscles

There are basically three methods of stretching.

1. Ballistic stretching: This type of stretching uses jumping type actions to stretch target muscle groups. Vinyasa Flow series are an example of ballistic stretching. This method is useful for "resetting" muscle length to that attained in a previous practice. Practicing the Sun Salutations in the morning is an example of this.

2. Passive stretching: This type of stretching involves the use of body weight, gravity, and synergist/agonist muscle groups to create a stretch. The body is placed into the position of stretch and held there for longer periods to allow the stretch receptors to "acclimate." This type of stretch affects the muscle spindle receptor in particular. Holding passive stretches for longer periods lengthens the noncontractile elements of the muscle, such as the fascial sheath.

3. Facilitated stretching: Also known as "PNF," or proprioceptive neuromuscular facilitation, involves briefly contracting the muscle targeted for stretch. This action stimulates the Golgi tendon organ stretch receptor, resulting in the spinal cord signaling the muscle to relax. The "slack" created by this response is then taken up by deepening the stretch.

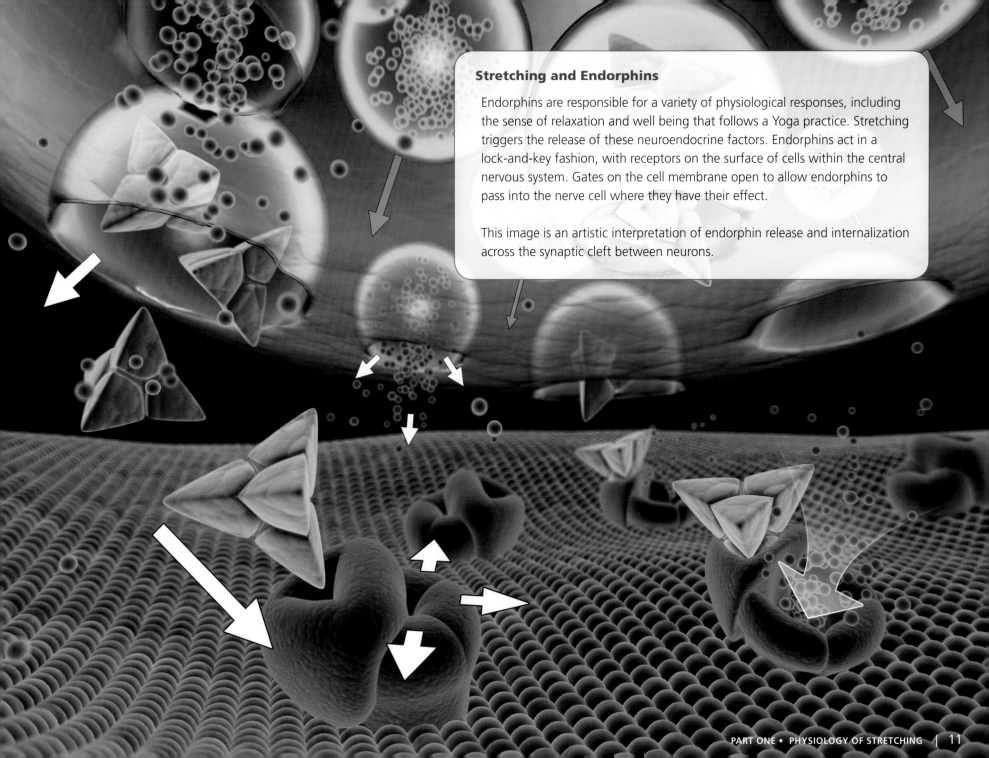

Stretching and Endorphins

Endorphins are responsible for a variety of physiological responses, including the sense of relaxation and well being that follows a Yoga practice. Stretching triggers the release of these neuroendocrine factors. Endorphins act in a lock-and-key fashion, with receptors on the surface of cells within the central nervous system. Gates on the cell membrane open to allow endorphins to pass into the nerve cell where they have their effect.

This image is an artistic interpretation of endorphin release and internalization across the synaptic cleft between neurons.

The Muscle Spindle Stretch Receptor

The muscle spindle stretch receptor is a modified muscle cell located in the "belly" of all skeletal muscles. It detects changes in length and tension within the muscle. Basically, when a muscle stretches, the muscle spindle sends a signal to the spinal cord, which then signals the muscle to contract and resist the stretch. This protects the muscle from over-stretching or tearing and is known as a "spinal cord reflex arc."

Never force the body into a stretch in Yoga, because this intensifies the firing of the muscle spindle, causing the muscle to contract. This mechanism can block deepening of the stretch. Rather, "dissolve" the blockages slowly by working with the spinal cord reflex arcs to decrease the reflex contraction of the muscle, and then go deeper into the pose.

The figure on the facing page illustrates the spinal cord reflex arc of the muscle spindle. A signal is sent from the muscle spindle receptor to the spinal cord. This signal is then relayed to the motor nerve via the spinal cord, signaling the muscle to contract and resist the stretch. This is a "primitive" reflex that occurs unconsciously in response to a biomechanical event, the stretching of a muscle. Holding a stretch for 30-60 seconds causes the muscle spindle to decrease its firing, and the muscle begins to relax. Backing part-way out of a stretch also decreases firing of the muscle spindle, relaxing the muscle and allowing a deeper stretch.

The following page uses the forward bend Uttanasana to describe a technique for "reassuring" the muscle spindle and decreasing its firing. This technique involves backing out part-way from the stretch for a few moments and then going into a deeper stretch. It may seem counterintuitive, but we can actually deepen a stretch by first backing off. This helps to decrease the reflex contraction of the muscles we are targeting for stretch.

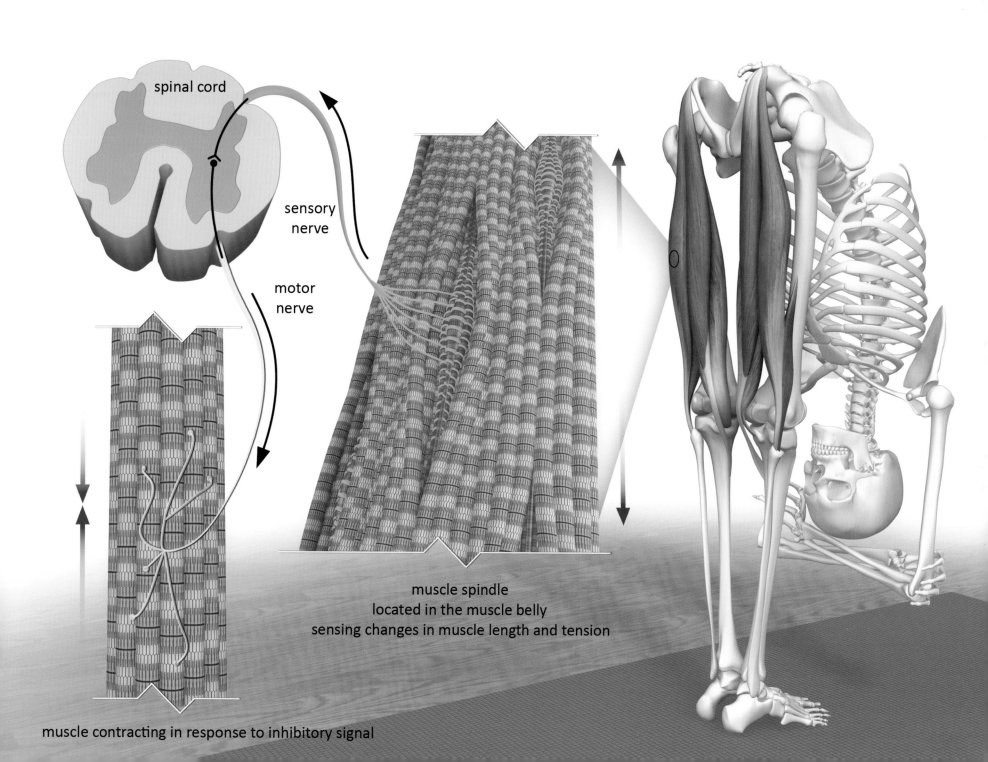

spinal cord

sensory
nerve

motor
nerve

muscle spindle
located in the muscle belly
sensing changes in muscle length and tension

muscle contracting in response to inhibitory signal

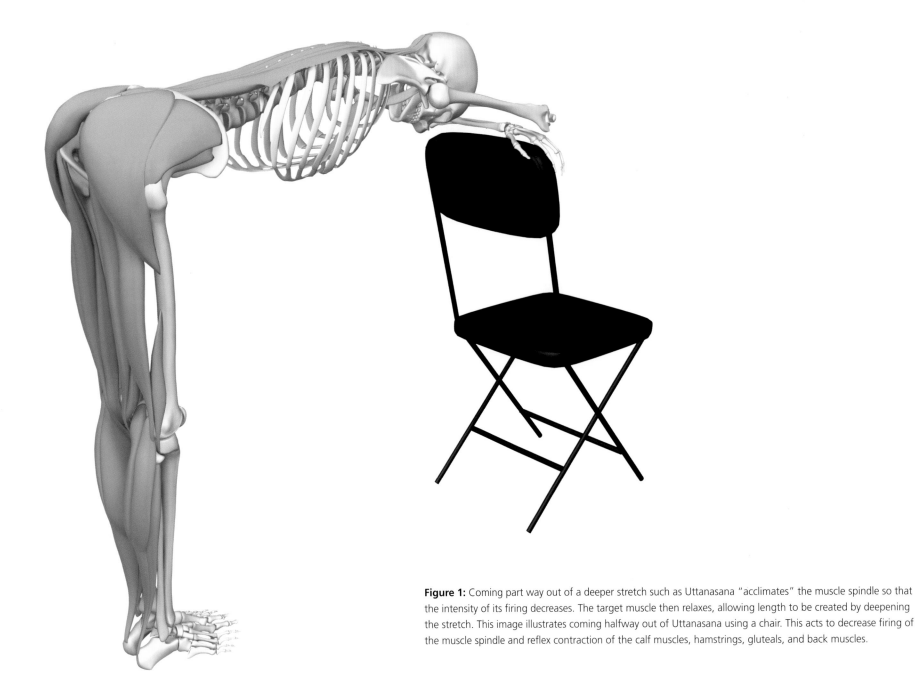

Figure 1: Coming part way out of a deeper stretch such as Uttanasana "acclimates" the muscle spindle so that the intensity of its firing decreases. The target muscle then relaxes, allowing length to be created by deepening the stretch. This image illustrates coming halfway out of Uttanasana using a chair. This acts to decrease firing of the muscle spindle and reflex contraction of the calf muscles, hamstrings, gluteals, and back muscles.

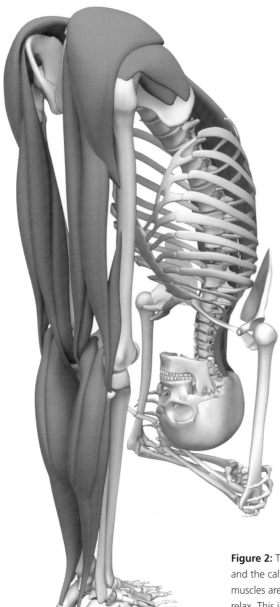

The muscle spindle in Uttanasana

Carefully bend forward in Uttanasana until you feel a moderate stretch. The muscle spindles of the hamstring, gluteus maximus, and erector spinae muscles will fire in response to this stretch and send a signal to the spinal cord. This is the first part of the reflex arc, with the muscle spindle connecting to the spine via the efferent nerve. The second part is the outgoing signal from the spinal cord via the afferent nerve to the muscle, signaling it to contract. The reflex contraction of the muscles of the back of the body—those being stretched—is part of what may prevent deepening in the posture Uttanasana.

The next step is to back off or "dissolve" reflex contraction of the stretched muscles by slightly relaxing the stretch. Chair Uttanasana is one way to acclimate the muscle spindle for forward bends, since lifting the torso decreases the intensity of the stretch of the muscles of the back body. Decreasing the stretch decreases the intensity of the firing of the muscle spindle, thus minimizing reflex contraction of the stretching muscles.

Hold this milder stretch for a few breaths. This quiets the muscle spindle stretch receptors and interrupts their 'alarm.' Once the muscle spindle adjusts to the milder stretch, contract the muscles at the front of the thigh to straighten the knees and deepen the pose.

Figure 2: The firing of the muscle spindle has decreased, and the calf muscles, hamstrings, gluteals, and back muscles are more relaxed, allowing the target muscles to relax. This image illustrates deepening of the stretch in Uttanasana.

Reciprocal Inhibition

The concept of the balanced Yin/Yang appears throughout the body. It is present in anatomy where the form of a joint fits its function. Consider again the shape of the hip and shoulder joints to see this concept in action.

The Biomechanical Yin/Yang

Muscles fall into two basic groups, depending on what we are doing at any given moment. For example, the quadriceps are the agonists for extending or straightening the knee. The hamstrings along the back of the thigh stretch when the knee extends and thus are the antagonists for this action. Conversely, the hamstrings become the agonist muscle when the knee bends, and the quadriceps become the antagonist. This is a biomechanical Yin/Yang.

Reciprocal Inhibition—A Physiological Yin/Yang

It makes sense that there would be a corresponding physiological Yin/Yang to make biomechanical processes such as bending and straightening the knee energy-efficient, i.e., when the agonist muscle contracts, its antagonist relaxes. This exists as the primitive spinal cord reflex known as reciprocal inhibition, meaning that muscles on one side of a joint relax to accommodate contraction on the other side of that joint. We can consciously access this reflex arc to deepen and improve our poses.

In Paschimottanasana, the quadriceps muscle along the front of the thigh is the agonist and the hamstring muscles along the back of the thigh are the antagonists. Contracting the quadriceps signals the hamstrings to relax. This takes place via the spinal cord. The nerve impulse that results in contraction of the quadriceps is called excitatory and the impulse to the hamstrings is called inhibitory.

Try this technique to get a bit deeper into this pose: firmly contract the quadriceps to straighten the knee, and note how the hamstring muscles relax. Apply it to different agonist/antagonist muscle groups in other poses. Note the added biomechanical benefit of improved bone alignment when you apply this technique.

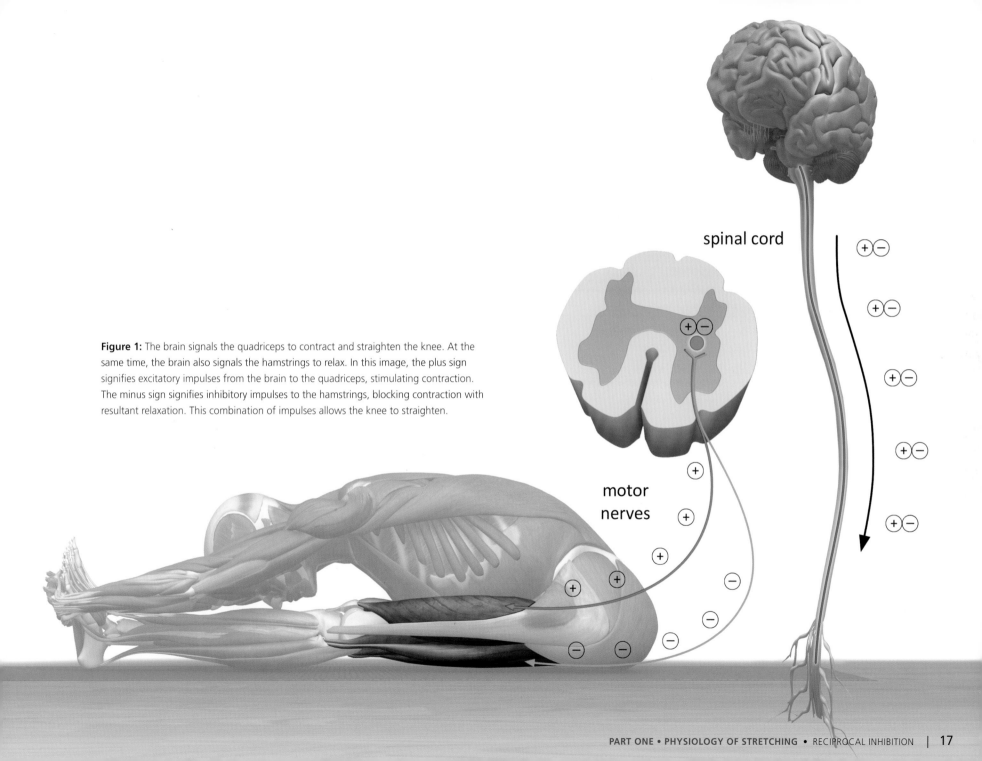

Figure 1: The brain signals the quadriceps to contract and straighten the knee. At the same time, the brain also signals the hamstrings to relax. In this image, the plus sign signifies excitatory impulses from the brain to the quadriceps, stimulating contraction. The minus sign signifies inhibitory impulses to the hamstrings, blocking contraction with resultant relaxation. This combination of impulses allows the knee to straighten.

spinal cord

motor
nerves

Golgi Tendon Organ

The Golgi tendon organ is a sensory receptor that is located where the muscle and tendon are joined. It detects changes in tension, and when tension increases, it signals the muscle to relax. This acts like a "circuit breaker" to prevent injury to the tendon when tension generated by the contracting muscle becomes too high. This contrasts with the muscle spindle receptor, which detects change in length and tension in the body of the muscle and signals the muscle to contract.

The Golgi tendon organ forms the basis for a phenomenon used by physical therapists and sports trainers known as proprioceptive neuromuscular facilitation, or "PNF." In PNF we temporarily contract a target muscle that we are stretching in order to stimulate the Golgi tendon organ. The Golgi tendon organ then signals the muscle to relax. This creates "slack" in the muscle that we can take up by going deeper into the stretch. This is known in physiology as the "relaxation response."

This may seem counterintuitive at first–contracting a muscle that we are trying to stretch; however, when applied carefully, this technique can be used to "dissolve" blocks and deepen poses. To understand the technique, we will look at lengthening the hamstrings in Janu Sirsasana. The technique is generally applied as follows:

1. First, take the muscle out to length. This establishes where the "set length" of the muscle is, the point that the brain recognizes as the end of the stretch.

2. Next, gently contract the target muscle. In this case, we are focusing on the hamstrings of the straight leg, so we attempt to bend the knee to create a contraction in the hamstrings (the action of the hamstrings is to bend the knee). I generally access this by slightly bending the knee and pressing the heel into the floor. This causes the hamstrings to contract.

3. Contract the muscle to no more than 20% of its maximum force and hold this for 8 to 10 seconds. Then relax for 1 breath.

4. Now, contract the antagonist muscles at the front of the thigh to take the target muscle out to a new "set" length. In this case, we contract the quadriceps to straighten the knee and bend deeper into the stretch of the hamstrings.

Hints and Cautions:

1. If you are new to Yoga, spend a few months conditioning your body first before using these powerful techniques to deepen stretches.

2. Remember that the Golgi tendon organ is there to protect the tendon from injury, but its ability to protect the tendon has limits. Never overdo it when using this technique. Never contract the target muscle more than about 20% of its maximum force.

3. The force generated by contracting muscles is transmitted to the joints. This is called the "joint reaction force," so you must always protect your joints by maintaining them in their natural alignment while stretching. If you experience joint pain, then back off from the stretch and stop.

4. Focus on one muscle group at a time, and limit your PNF stretching to one pose in a practice session. Do no more than 2 to 3 cycles of the stretch described above.

5. Allow ample time (48 hours) for recovery before repeating this technique.

6. Always practice under the guidance of an experienced and qualified teacher.

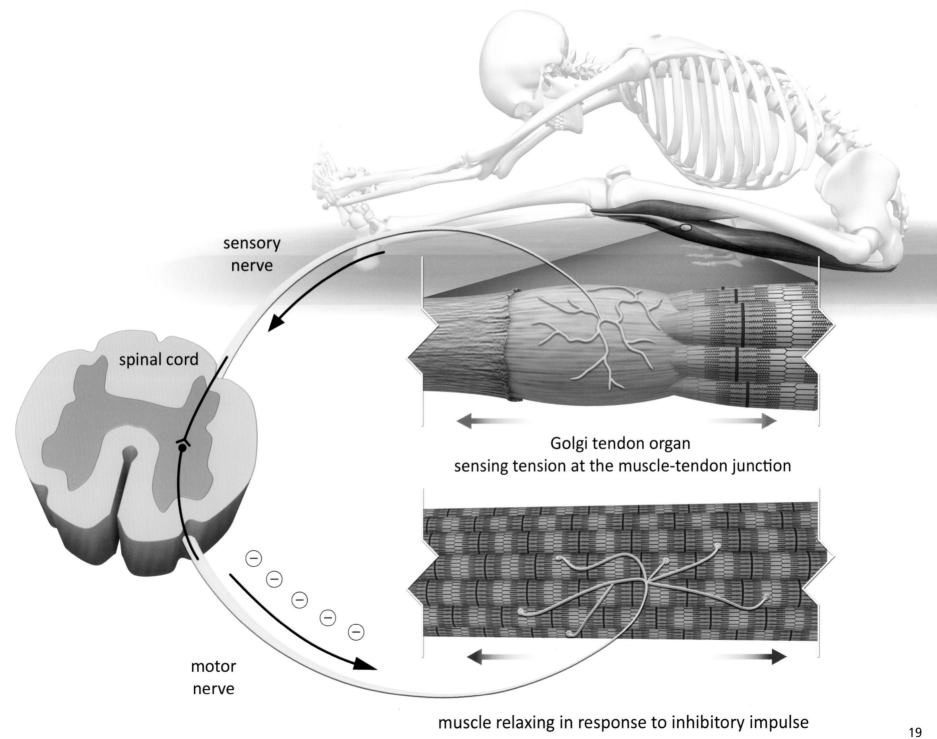

sensory
nerve

spinal cord

Golgi tendon organ
sensing tension at the muscle-tendon junction

motor
nerve

muscle relaxing in response to inhibitory impulse

The Golgi Tendon Organ and Facilitated Stretching

Attempting to pull the hands apart in Gomukhasana increases the tension at the muscle-tendon junctions of the upper extremities. This affects the muscle-tendon junctions of the infraspinatus and teres minor muscles of the rotator cuff, as well as the front portion of the deltoid and the upper pectoralis (in the lower arm of the pose). In the upper arm of the pose, the increased tension is felt in the subscapularis muscle of the rotator cuff as well as the latissimus dorsi and teres major.

The firing of the Golgi tendon organ in response to this tension results in the spinal cord signaling these muscles to relax. This relaxation response persists for a brief period, even after release of the tension created by pulling the hands apart. The pose can then be deepened by moving the hands closer together and taking up the slack created by the relaxation response.

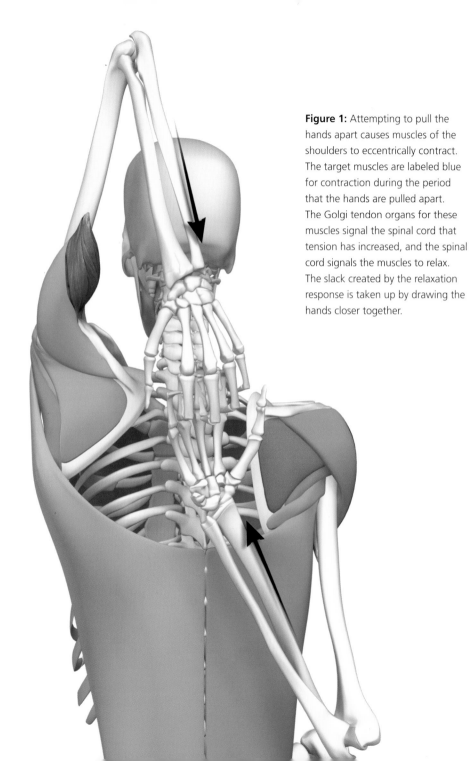

Figure 1: Attempting to pull the hands apart causes muscles of the shoulders to eccentrically contract. The target muscles are labeled blue for contraction during the period that the hands are pulled apart. The Golgi tendon organs for these muscles signal the spinal cord that tension has increased, and the spinal cord signals the muscles to relax. The slack created by the relaxation response is taken up by drawing the hands closer together.

20

The back leg in modified Lunge Pose illustrates facilitated stretching of the hip flexors. The knee of the back leg and the foot of the front leg are both fixed on the mat. This means that the force generated by contracting the back leg flexors will manifest as tension at the muscle-tendon junctions of these muscles. The Golgi tendon organs of the hip flexors will send their signal to the spinal cord which, in turn, will signal the flexors to relax. The slack created by the relaxation response is then taken up by going deeper into the lunge.

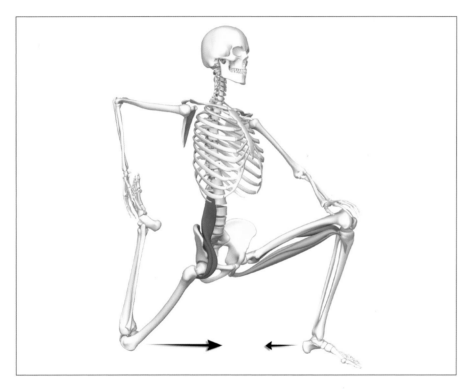

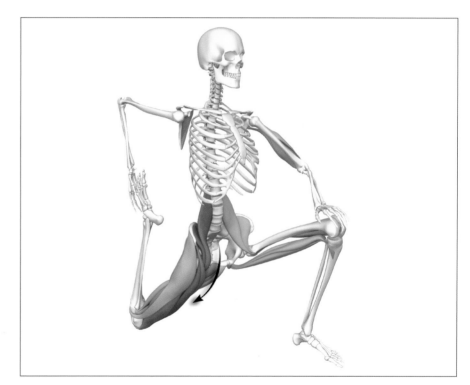

Figure 1: The psoas is a flexor of the hip that has been isolated for this illustration. The hip is taken into extension, stretching the psoas. Attempting to drag the back knee toward the front foot causes the stretched psoas to contract eccentrically, stimulating the Golgi tendon organs at its muscle-tendon junction. This tension can be increased by contracting the front leg hamstrings and attempting to drag the front foot toward the back knee. The front foot is fixed, so the force of this contraction is transmitted to the back leg psoas, increasing the firing of the Golgi tendon organs of that muscle.

Figure 2: The slack in the flexor group is then taken up by deepening the pose. Activating the front leg psoas flexes the hip, while the hamstrings bend the knee. Pressing down on the front knee with the hand lifts the trunk. All of these actions deepen the pose and lengthen the hip flexors of the back leg.

Combining Biomechanics and Physiology in Stretching

Here we use Janu Sirsasana to illustrate stretching the hamstrings by moving their origins and insertions in combination with techniques we have gained from knowledge of the muscle spindle, reciprocal inhibition, and the Golgi tendon organ.

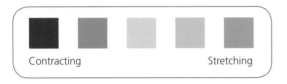

Contracting   Stretching

1. Take the general form of the pose to apply a moderate stretch to the hamstring muscles of the straight leg. This stimulates the muscle spindle to fire, resulting in reflex contraction of the hamstrings.

2. Bend the knee to lighten the stretch of the hamstrings, releasing their insertion on the lower leg. Hold this relaxed position for 2 or 3 breaths as the muscle spindle accomodates to the lighter stretch.

3. Now that the firing of the muscle spindle has decreased, contract the quadriceps to straighten the knee and draw the hamstrings out to length, moving the insertion at the knee away from the origin. This action signals the hamstrings to further relax via reciprocal inhibition.

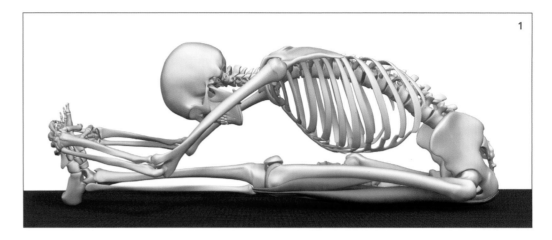

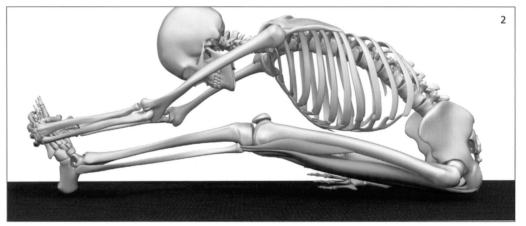

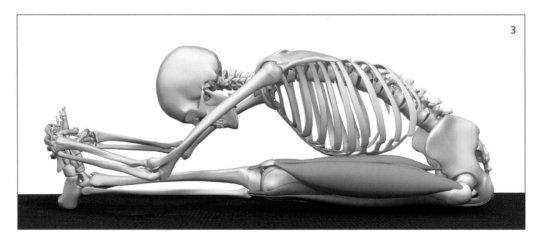

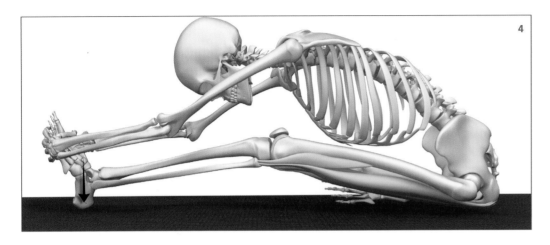

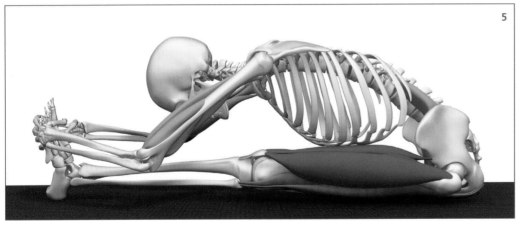

4. Attempt to press the heel into the ground by contracting the hamstrings. This increases tension at the muscle-tendon junction and stimulates the Golgi tendon organ to fire. The spinal cord then signals the hamstrings to relax.

5. Contract the quadriceps to straighten the knee and move the insertion of the hamstrings away from the origin. Straightening the knee takes up the "slack" created by the relaxation response. Contracting the quadriceps creates reciprocal inhibition, further relaxing the hamstrings. The psoas tilts the pelvis forward, moving the hamstring origin away from the insertion. Bending the elbows by contracting the biceps bends the trunk forward, deepening the pose.

Muscle Awakening

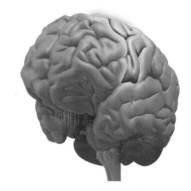

The motor cortex highlighted here in blue.

Certain muscles become active early in life for movements that we perform regularly. One such muscle is the psoas, a core postural muscle of the pelvis and lumbar spine. We begin using the psoas at around 8 months of age, when we first flex the trunk to sit up. The brain quickly perceives that this is an activity we will do regularly and creates circuitry within the motor cortex to perform this task unconsciously. This is because the body seeks to conserve energy. Thinking about something expends energy. Imagine if we had to think about each step before taking it! In fact, we use our postural muscles so frequently that we "forget" how to activate them consciously.

Yoga postures place new demands on the body that are different from activities of daily living (such as sitting up or walking), and they activate our conscious awareness of dormant muscles such as the psoas. Once re-awakened, we can consciously bring these muscles into play for new tasks. For example, we can use the newly awakened psoas to deepen and improve the same Yoga postures we used to awaken it.

This chapter focuses on the psoas muscle. This is a polyarticular muscle that originates from the lumbar spine, crosses over the pelvis, and inserts on the inside of the femur. As a consequence, contracting this important muscle can stabilize the lumbar spine, tilt the pelvis, and flex the femur. One of the keys to effectively practicing Yoga is to activate the prime movers of a given region—those muscles that most efficiently create the form of the pose. For example, in the pose Trikonasana, it is possible to flex the hip by simply bending over the leg using the force of gravity. Trikonasana becomes more precise and beneficial, however, by activating the main flexor of the hip, the psoas.

Body Clairvoyance

The word clairvoyance means "seeing clearly." Body clairvoyance refers to the ability of the awakened body to anticipate an action and use the most efficient muscles to accomplish it. Practicing Yoga creates this type of phenomenon, a feeling of "knowing" what to do. As the energy channels open, the path of the cosmos becomes clear.

Yoga poses can be combined to sequentially activate different parts of the body. The standing poses in this book are arranged in just such a sequence, targeting the psoas and core muscles.

When the brain sees a combination of actions like The Psoas Awakening Series, it begins to automatically use the muscle in unrelated actions. This is analogous to running up a flight of stairs. The first steps are taken consciously, but once we get going, we ascend unconsciously (and rhythmically). We see this same phenomenon with professional athletes when they practice fundamental movements in their sport and then spontaneously "cut loose" on the field. Put another way, consciously awakening the dormant psoas muscle causes us to then use it unconsciously in new tasks.

I demonstrate this phenomenon in my workshops by finishing the Psoas Awakening Series with an inversion, such as full arm balance. Students regularly report a sensation of rock solid stability in their pose. This comes from the unconscious brain automatically activating the newly awakened psoas and stabilizing the pelvis in a new task. Experience this for yourself by practicing an unrelated pose at the end of the series.

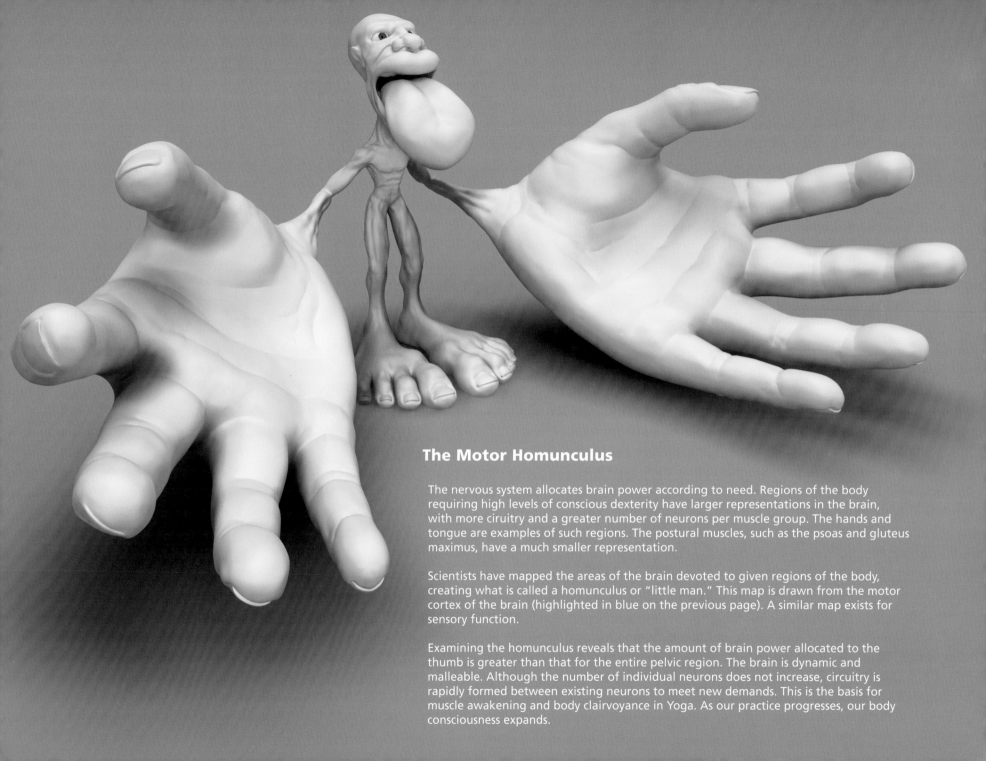

The Motor Homunculus

The nervous system allocates brain power according to need. Regions of the body requiring high levels of conscious dexterity have larger representations in the brain, with more ciruitry and a greater number of neurons per muscle group. The hands and tongue are examples of such regions. The postural muscles, such as the psoas and gluteus maximus, have a much smaller representation.

Scientists have mapped the areas of the brain devoted to given regions of the body, creating what is called a homunculus or "little man." This map is drawn from the motor cortex of the brain (highlighted in blue on the previous page). A similar map exists for sensory function.

Examining the homunculus reveals that the amount of brain power allocated to the thumb is greater than that for the entire pelvic region. The brain is dynamic and malleable. Although the number of individual neurons does not increase, circuitry is rapidly formed between existing neurons to meet new demands. This is the basis for muscle awakening and body clairvoyance in Yoga. As our practice progresses, our body consciousness expands.

Awakening the Psoas

This chapter presents a synergistic combination of standing poses that effectively activates and re-awakens the psoas muscle. We accomplish this by first contracting the psoas in poses that face forward, then in poses that face the side. We complete the series with the twisting postures. In this way, we can sequentially "walk" activation of the psoas around the muscle, progressively awakening it in a slightly different manner with each pose. This creates the phenomenon of body clairvoyance where the brain "anticipates" actions where using the psoas would be beneficial (other Yoga poses) and automatically engages it for that activity.

Remember that, since this muscle is usually "hidden" in the unconscious part of the brain, we must first isolate it in each pose and bring it back into conscious awareness. Isometric contraction is one way to isolate and awaken a dormant muscle. This means that the muscle is activated, but instead of being allowed to lengthen or shorten, it is held at a constant length. This technique requires an understanding of the action of the various muscles. For example, the psoas acts to flex the hip, i.e., contracting the psoas either bends the trunk forward or draws the knee up. Isolate and hone your awareness of the psoas by attempting to flex the trunk or lift the leg. Placing the arm on the knee can be used to accentuate this by resisting the action. To better understand this, refer to the diagram of Trikonasana in Figure 1.

The following pages illustrate a short series of poses that can be used to isolate and awaken the psoas, with insets showing isometric contraction. The full Psoas Awakening Series is illustrated in the standing pose section.

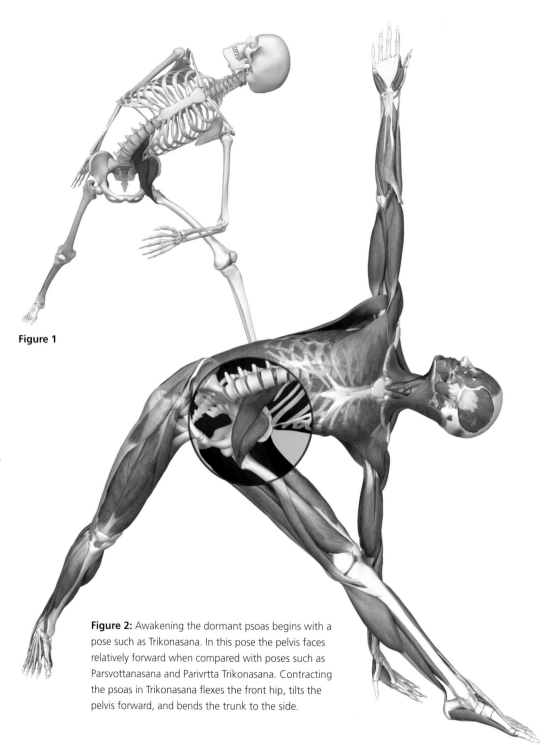

Figure 1

Figure 2: Awakening the dormant psoas begins with a pose such as Trikonasana. In this pose the pelvis faces relatively forward when compared with poses such as Parsvottanasana and Parivrtta Trikonasana. Contracting the psoas in Trikonasana flexes the front hip, tilts the pelvis forward, and bends the trunk to the side.

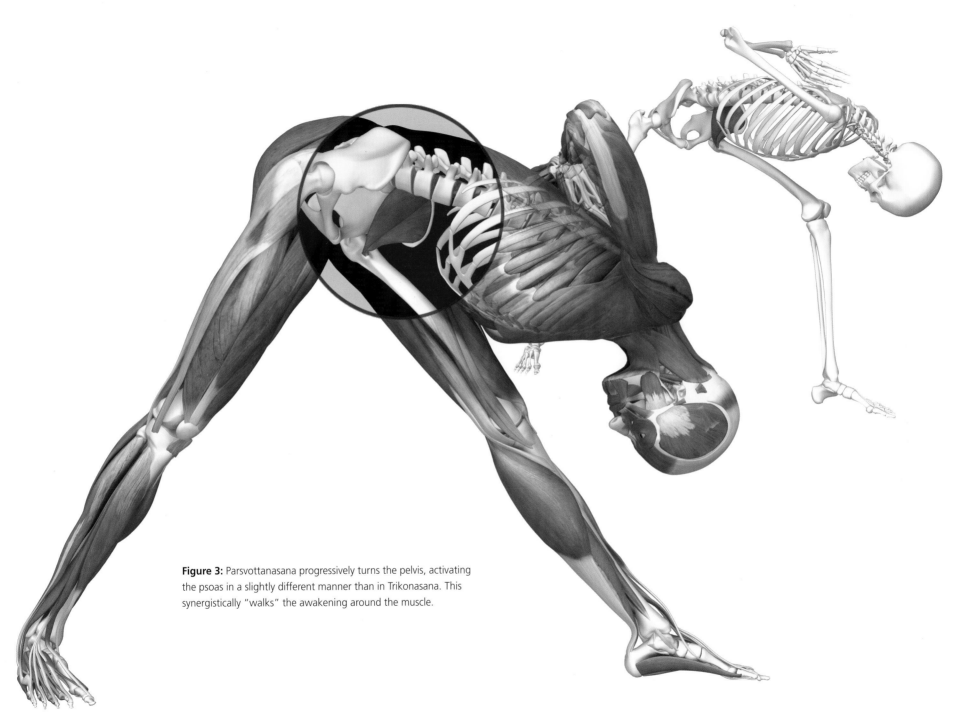

Figure 3: Parsvottanasana progressively turns the pelvis, activating the psoas in a slightly different manner than in Trikonasana. This synergistically "walks" the awakening around the muscle.

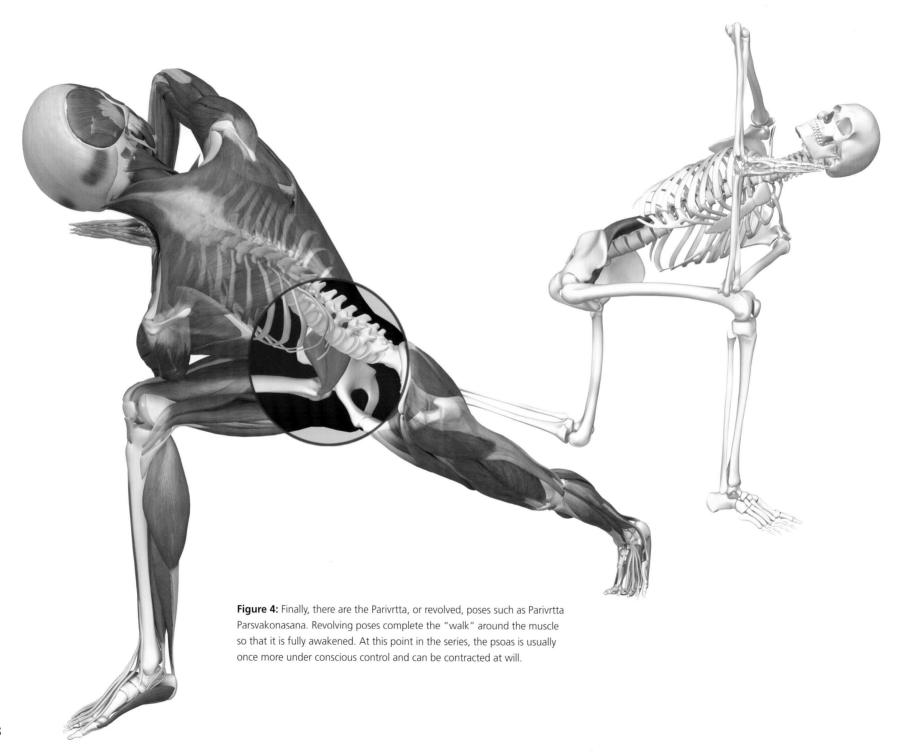

Figure 4: Finally, there are the Parivrtta, or revolved, poses such as Parivrtta Parsvakonasana. Revolving poses complete the "walk" around the muscle so that it is fully awakened. At this point in the series, the psoas is usually once more under conscious control and can be contracted at will.

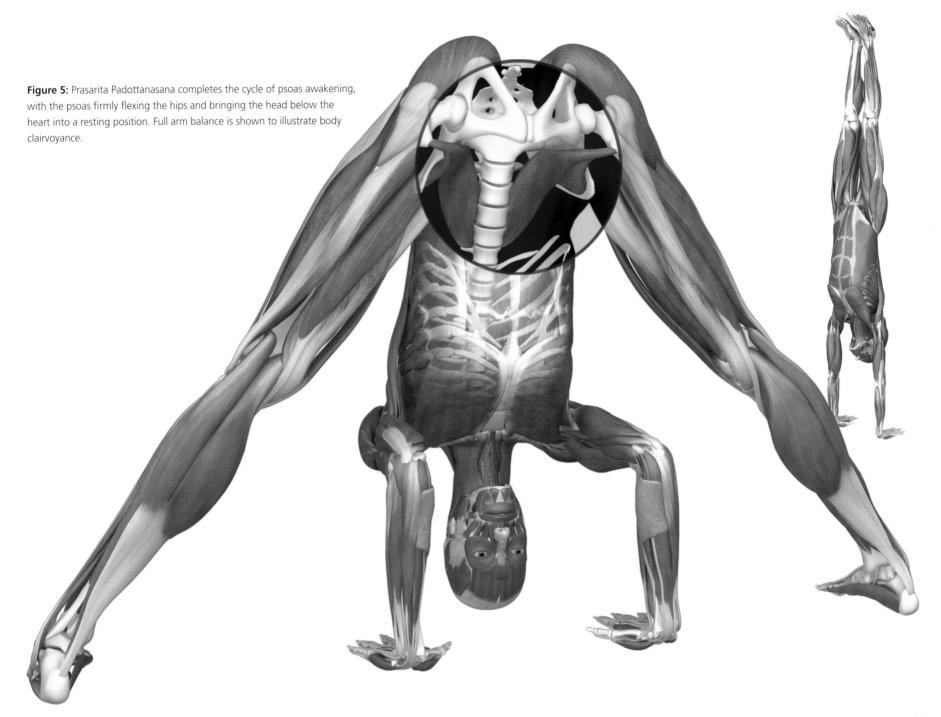

Figure 5: Prasarita Padottanasana completes the cycle of psoas awakening, with the psoas firmly flexing the hips and bringing the head below the heart into a resting position. Full arm balance is shown to illustrate body clairvoyance.

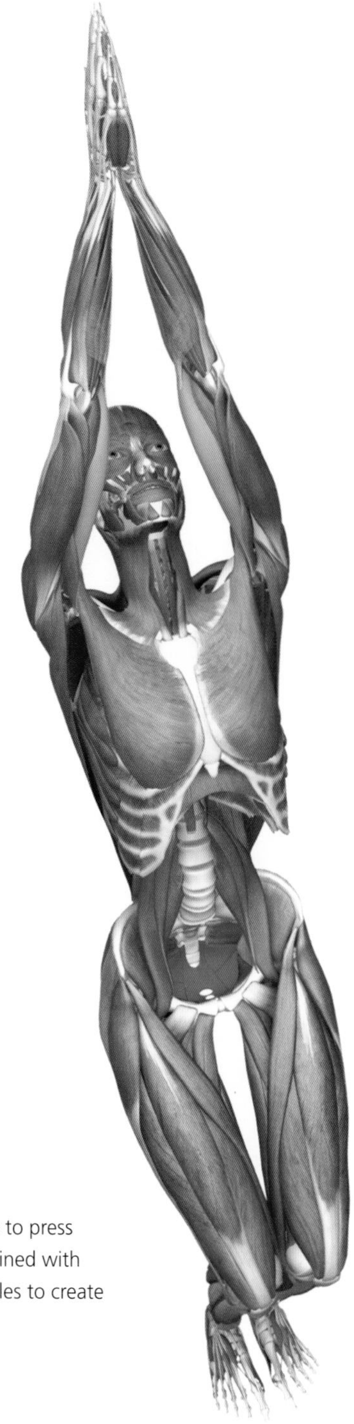

Recruitment and Bandhas

Gaining awareness of a muscle such as the psoas is relatively straightforward. This is because the psoas can be isolated and activated by flexing the hip. Isometric contraction of the psoas effectively brings it under conscious control.

Other muscles, such as those comprising the pelvic diaphragm, are more deeply buried in the unconscious and, by virtue of their more subtle actions, are more difficult to isolate. The technique of recruitment can be used to bring about awareness and control of such muscle groups. Recruitment is a process whereby one contracts an easily accessed muscle group while simultaneously contracting "hidden" muscles, such as those of the pelvic floor.

Physicians use this technique when examining the integrity of the deep tendon reflexes. For example, in a patient with a weak knee jerk reflex, the physician may ask them to grasp their hands together and attempt to pull them apart and then tap the patellar tendon. This creates a rapid stretch in the quadriceps muscle and stimulates the muscle spindle receptor. The result is a signal to the quadriceps to contract. Combining the patellar tap with pulling the hands apart causes the quadriceps to contract more forcefully. This technique is known as recruitment.

Figure 1: Contracting the biceps to press the hands together can be combined with contracting the pelvic floor muscles to create a more powerful Mula Bandha.

Bandha is a Sanskrit word meaning "lock" or "bind." In the Bandhas, we contract certain muscle groups to create an energy "lock" in the body. Classically, this refers to the three major Bandhas—Mula Bandha, Udyana Bandha, and Jalandhara Bandha. Mula Bandha involves contracting the muscles of the pelvic floor to lift and tone the pelvic organs and illuminate the first and second Chakras.

Recruitment is a particularly useful aid for awakening the difficult-to-access muscles of the perineum and pelvic diaphragm that create Mula Bandha. It can be performed in virtually any Yoga pose by contracting a muscle group that is easy to access and combining this action with contracting the muscles of the perineum (also known as the Kegel maneuver). Try this by combining pressing the hands together in Utkatasana and contracting the muscles of the pelvic floor. Notice how much more powerful Mula Bandha feels. Figures 1 and 2 illustrate this process in the poses Utkatasana and Marichyasana III.

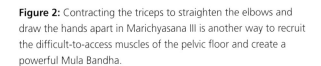

Figure 2: Contracting the triceps to straighten the elbows and draw the hands apart in Marichyasana III is another way to recruit the difficult-to-access muscles of the pelvic floor and create a powerful Mula Bandha.

Zen Buddhism and Awakening: The Ten Bull Pictures

The Ten Bull Pictures is a Buddhist parable that illustrates the stages of awakening to hidden potential. The story uses a series of pictures to tell the story of a student seeking, finding, and integrating knowledge of the self. The images use a bull as the symbol of this knowledge. The bull itself eventually disappears, but the knowledge remains and becomes part of the individual.

Practicing Yoga follows a similar sequence. Yoga is the yoke that connects us to the bull. Hatha Yoga re-awakens body consciousness and re-establishes the mind/body connection. The Ten Bull Pictures is a metaphor for this process.

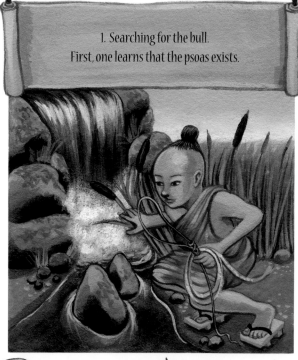

1. Searching for the bull.
First, one learns that the psoas exists.

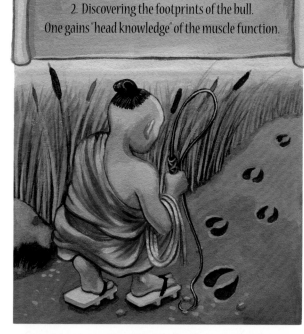

2. Discovering the footprints of the bull.
One gains "head knowledge" of the muscle function.

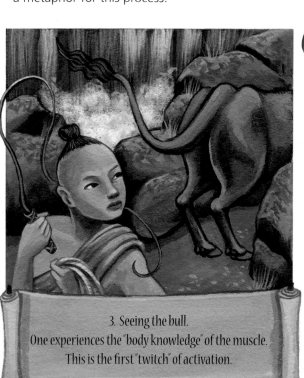

3. Seeing the bull.
One experiences the "body knowledge" of the muscle. This is the first "twitch" of activation.

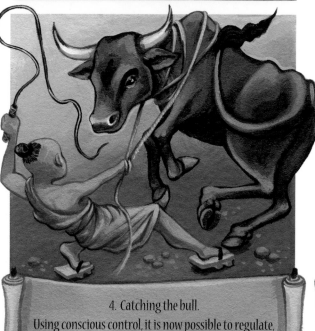

4. Catching the bull.
Using conscious control, it is now possible to regulate, in rough fashion, the force of contraction.

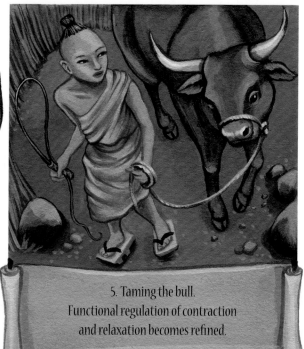

5. Taming the bull.
Functional regulation of contraction and relaxation becomes refined.

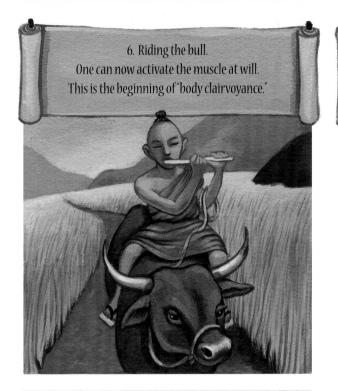

6. Riding the bull.
One can now activate the muscle at will.
This is the beginning of "body clairvoyance."

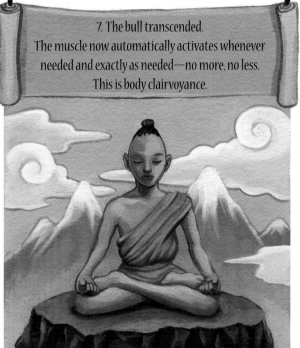

7. The bull transcended.
The muscle now automatically activates whenever
needed and exactly as needed—no more, no less.
This is body clairvoyance.

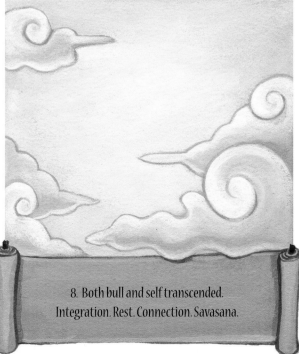

8. Both bull and self transcended.
Integration. Rest. Connection. Savasana.

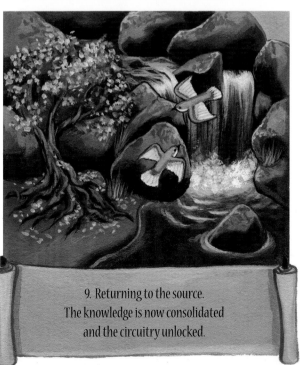

9. Returning to the source.
The knowledge is now consolidated
and the circuitry unlocked.

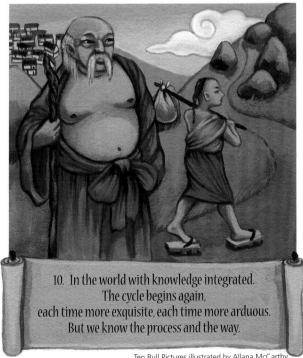

10. In the world with knowledge integrated.
The cycle begins again,
each time more exquisite, each time more arduous.
But we know the process and the way.

Ten Bull Pictures illustrated by Allana McCarthy.

Part Two: Practice

Preparatory Poses

Preparatory poses apply a targeted stretch to a specific region of the body, such as the shoulders or hips, focusing on an elemental movement such as flexion of the shoulders or rotation of the hips. The goal is to create increased range of motion in an area of the body, then integrate this into the poses.

The preparatory poses can be used as a general stretch prior to or during practice, or to prepare the body for a specific pose. For example, deconstructing Eka Pada Rajakapotasana I (Pigeon Pose) reveals that the front hip is turning outward, the back hip is extending, and the shoulders are fully flexing over the head (Figures 1, 2, and 3).

The following pages illustrate several preparatory poses that increase the range of motion for these regions of the body, preparing for Eka Pada Rajakapotasana I. Additional examples of preparatory poses conclude this chapter.

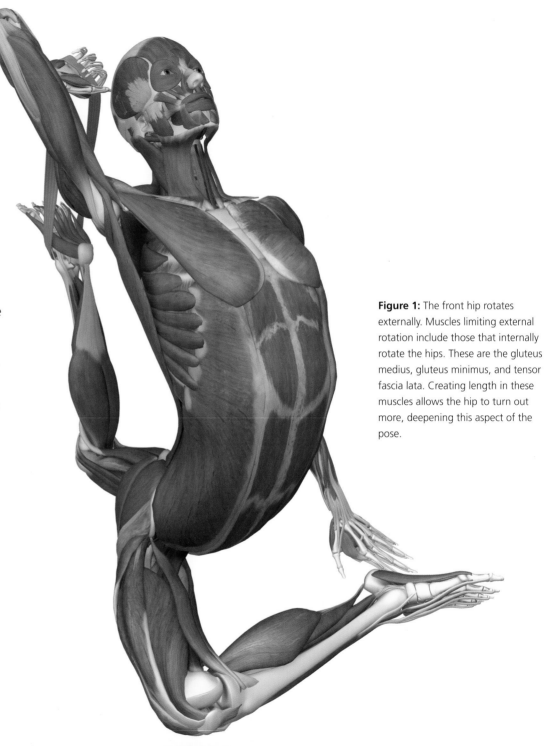

Figure 1: The front hip rotates externally. Muscles limiting external rotation include those that internally rotate the hips. These are the gluteus medius, gluteus minimus, and tensor fascia lata. Creating length in these muscles allows the hip to turn out more, deepening this aspect of the pose.

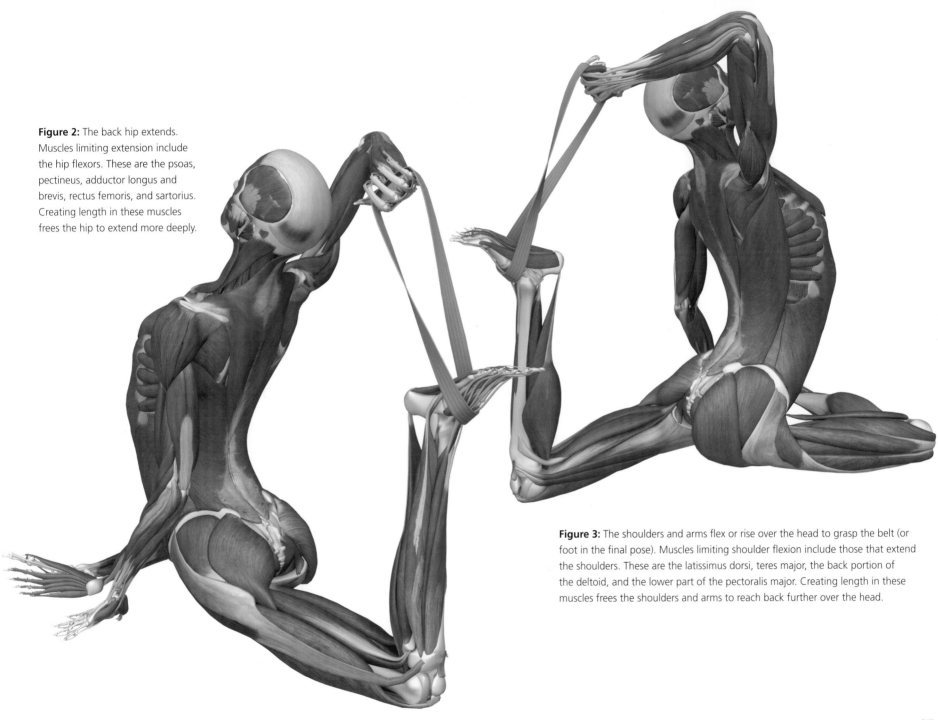

Figure 2: The back hip extends. Muscles limiting extension include the hip flexors. These are the psoas, pectineus, adductor longus and brevis, rectus femoris, and sartorius. Creating length in these muscles frees the hip to extend more deeply.

Figure 3: The shoulders and arms flex or rise over the head to grasp the belt (or foot in the final pose). Muscles limiting shoulder flexion include those that extend the shoulders. These are the latissimus dorsi, teres major, the back portion of the deltoid, and the lower part of the pectoralis major. Creating length in these muscles frees the shoulders and arms to reach back further over the head.

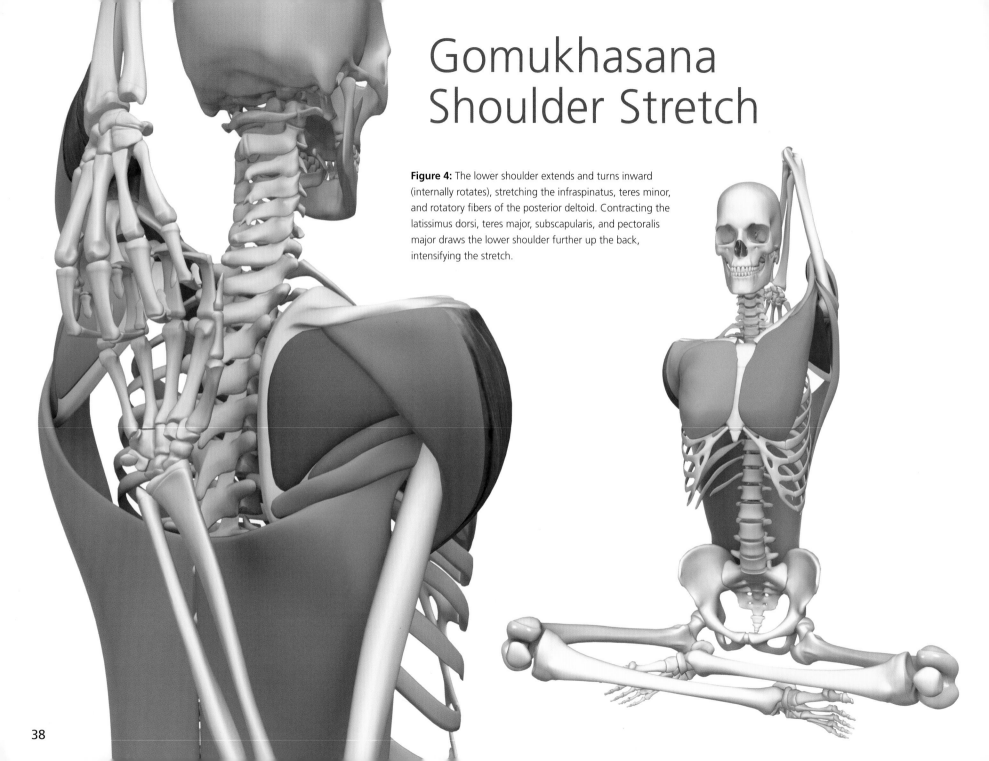

Gomukhasana Shoulder Stretch

Figure 4: The lower shoulder extends and turns inward (internally rotates), stretching the infraspinatus, teres minor, and rotatory fibers of the posterior deltoid. Contracting the latissimus dorsi, teres major, subscapularis, and pectoralis major draws the lower shoulder further up the back, intensifying the stretch.

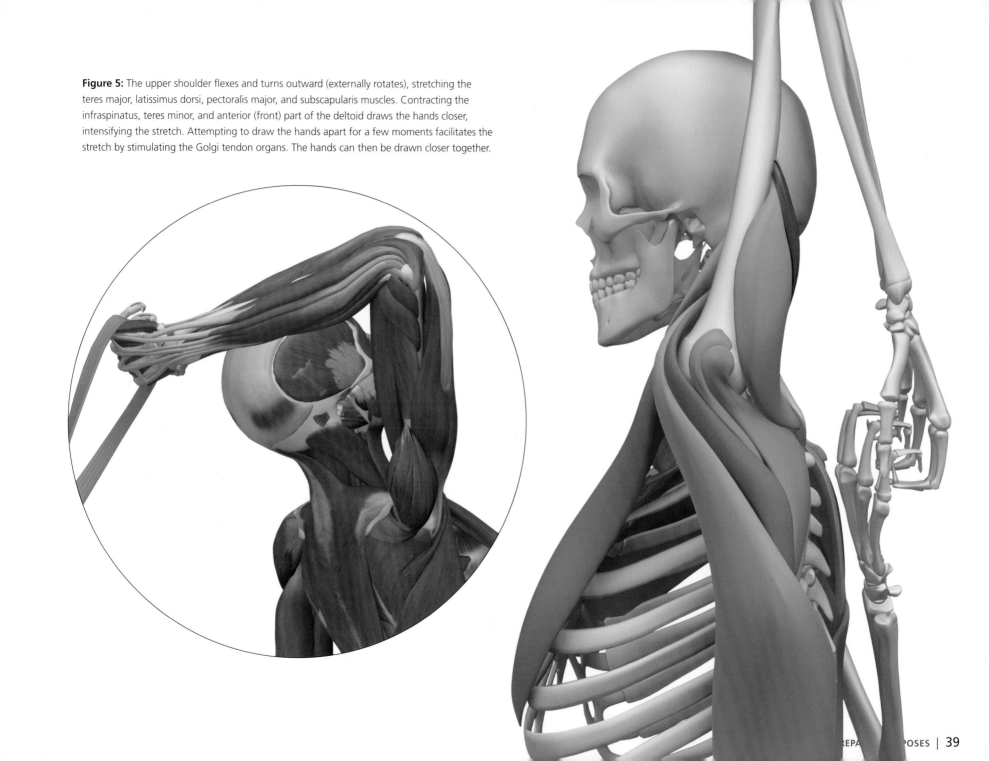

Figure 5: The upper shoulder flexes and turns outward (externally rotates), stretching the teres major, latissimus dorsi, pectoralis major, and subscapularis muscles. Contracting the infraspinatus, teres minor, and anterior (front) part of the deltoid draws the hands closer, intensifying the stretch. Attempting to draw the hands apart for a few moments facilitates the stretch by stimulating the Golgi tendon organs. The hands can then be drawn closer together.

Hip Internal Rotator and Extensor Stretch

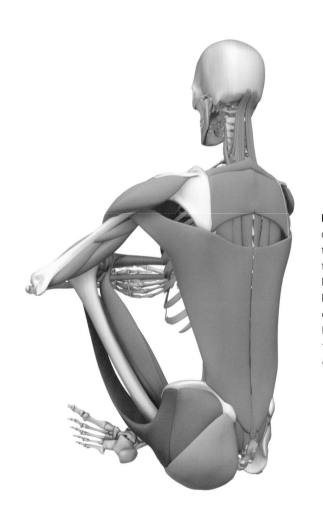

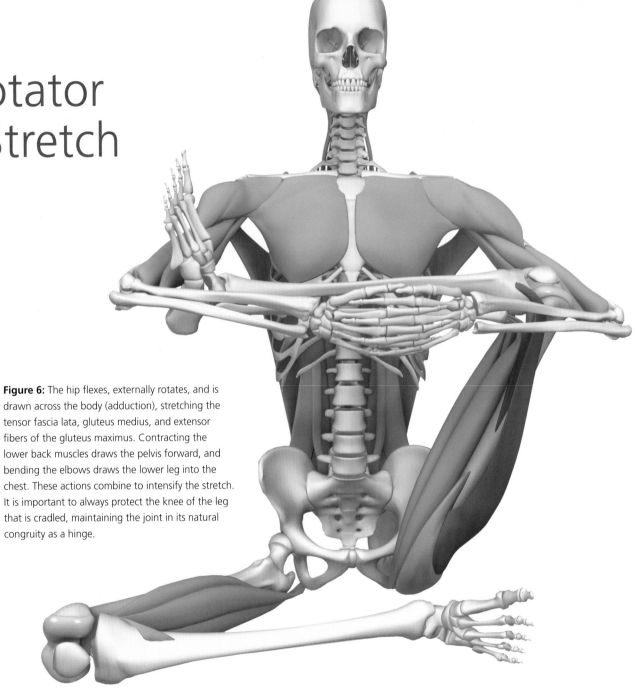

Figure 6: The hip flexes, externally rotates, and is drawn across the body (adduction), stretching the tensor fascia lata, gluteus medius, and extensor fibers of the gluteus maximus. Contracting the lower back muscles draws the pelvis forward, and bending the elbows draws the lower leg into the chest. These actions combine to intensify the stretch. It is important to always protect the knee of the leg that is cradled, maintaining the joint in its natural congruity as a hinge.

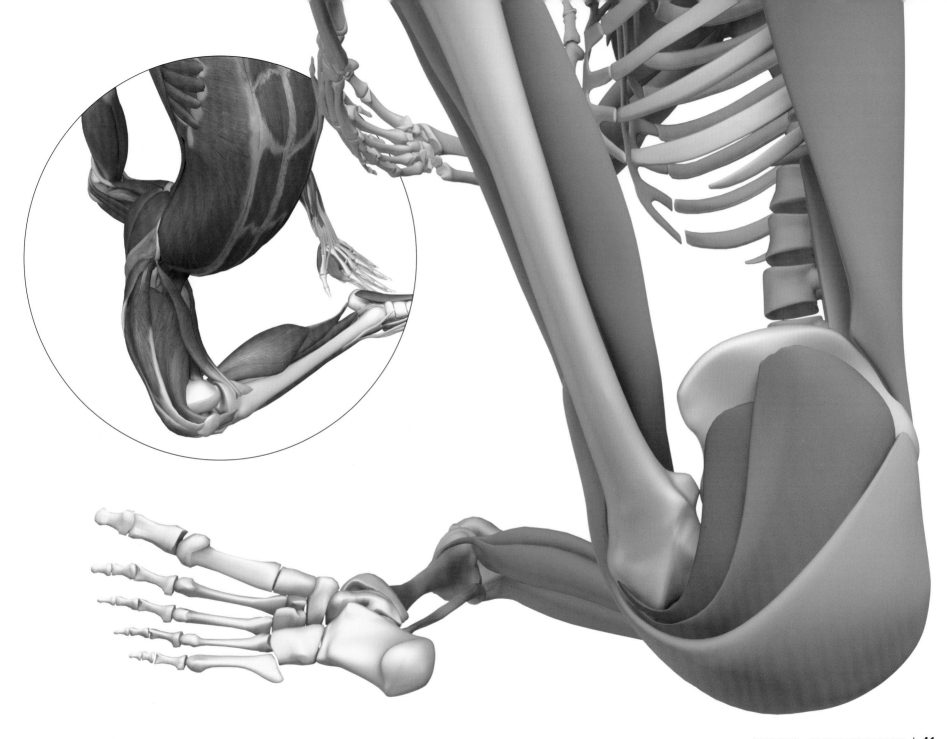

Psoas and Quadriceps Stretch

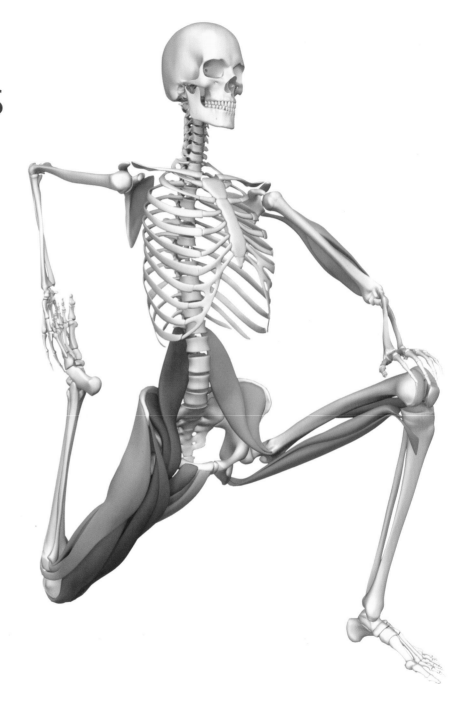

Figure 7: The back hip extends and the knees flex, stretching the psoas, pectineus, rectus femoris, sartorius, and adductors longus and magnus. Contracting the back leg gluteals intensifies the stretch of the hip flexors. Bending the front knee, flexing the front hip, and lifting the torso also intensifies the stretch. Attempting to draw the back knee toward the front foot for a few moments creates a facilitated stretch, stimulating the Golgi tendon organs of the muscles that are stretching.

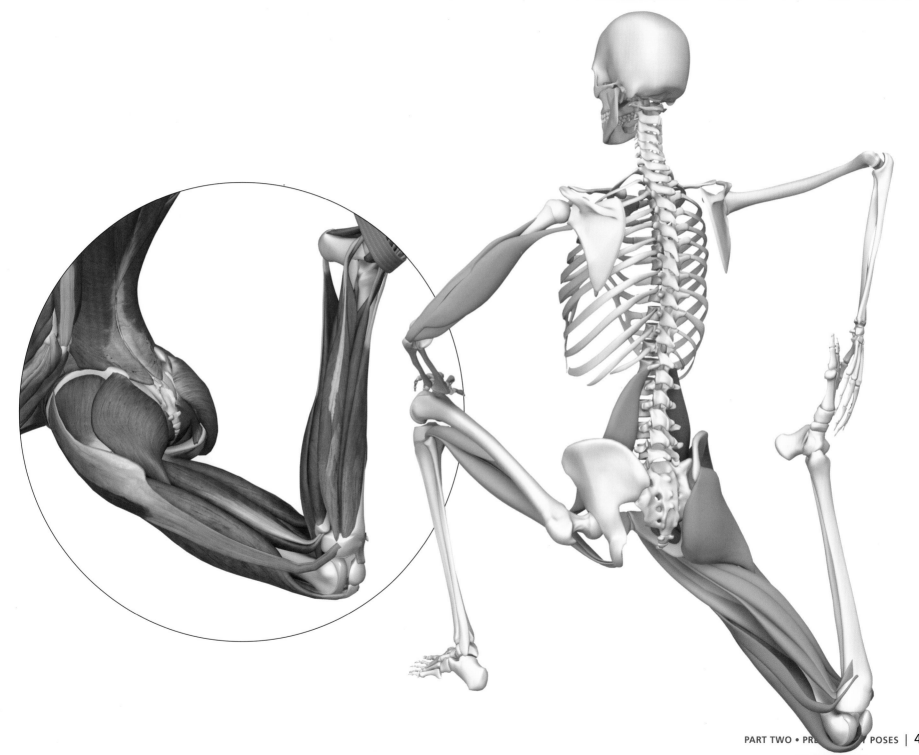

Garudasana Arms and Shoulders

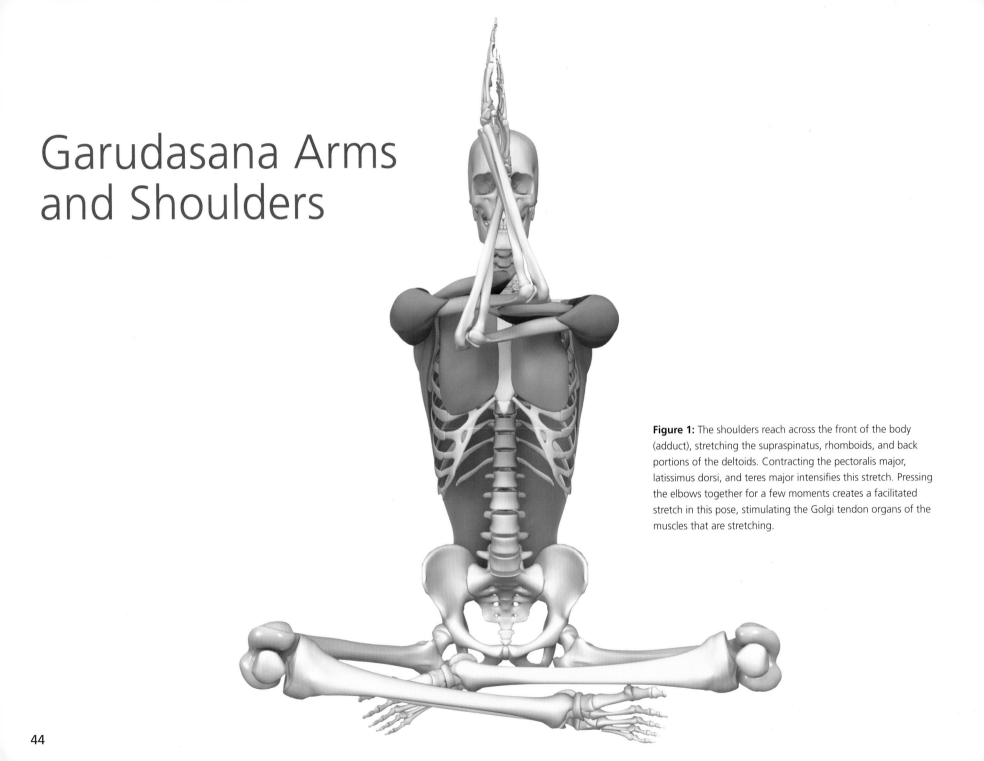

Figure 1: The shoulders reach across the front of the body (adduct), stretching the supraspinatus, rhomboids, and back portions of the deltoids. Contracting the pectoralis major, latissimus dorsi, and teres major intensifies this stretch. Pressing the elbows together for a few moments creates a facilitated stretch in this pose, stimulating the Golgi tendon organs of the muscles that are stretching.

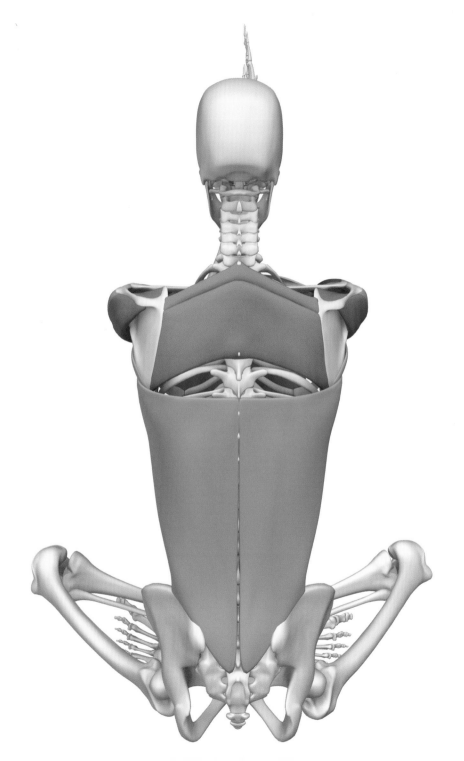

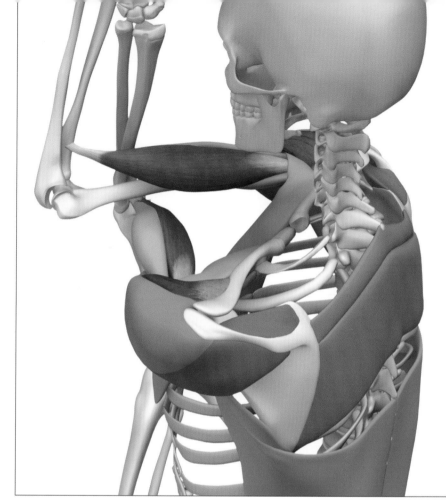

Figure 2: The shoulders reach across the front of the body (adduct), stretching the back portions of the deltoids, supraspinatus, and rhomboids. Contracting the pectoralis major, latissimus dorsi, and teres major intensifies this stretch. Pressing the elbows together for a few moments creates a facilitated stretch in this pose, stimulating the Golgi tendon organs of the muscles that are stretching.

Shoulder Extensor Stretch (with chair)

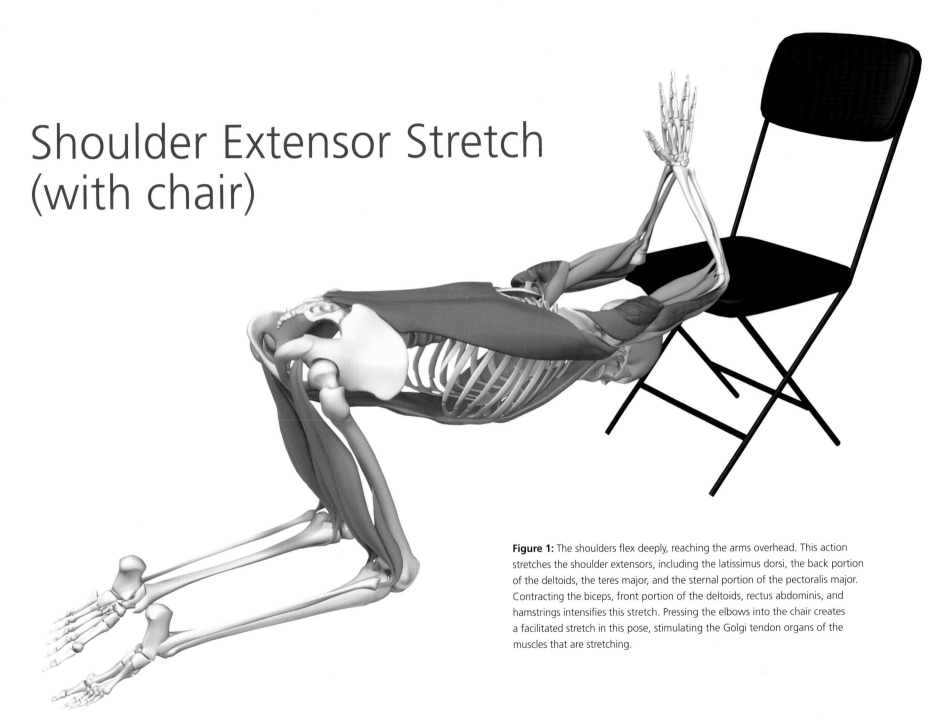

Figure 1: The shoulders flex deeply, reaching the arms overhead. This action stretches the shoulder extensors, including the latissimus dorsi, the back portion of the deltoids, the teres major, and the sternal portion of the pectoralis major. Contracting the biceps, front portion of the deltoids, rectus abdominis, and hamstrings intensifies this stretch. Pressing the elbows into the chair creates a facilitated stretch in this pose, stimulating the Golgi tendon organs of the muscles that are stretching.

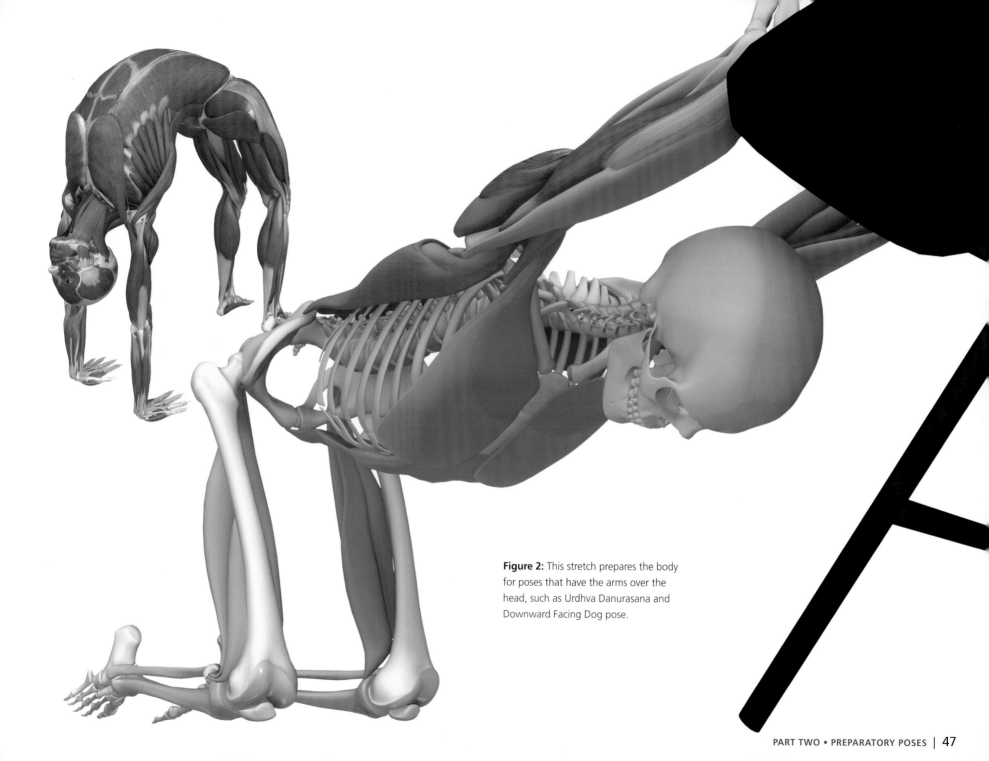

Figure 2: This stretch prepares the body for poses that have the arms over the head, such as Urdhva Danurasana and Downward Facing Dog pose.

Shoulder Flexor Stretch

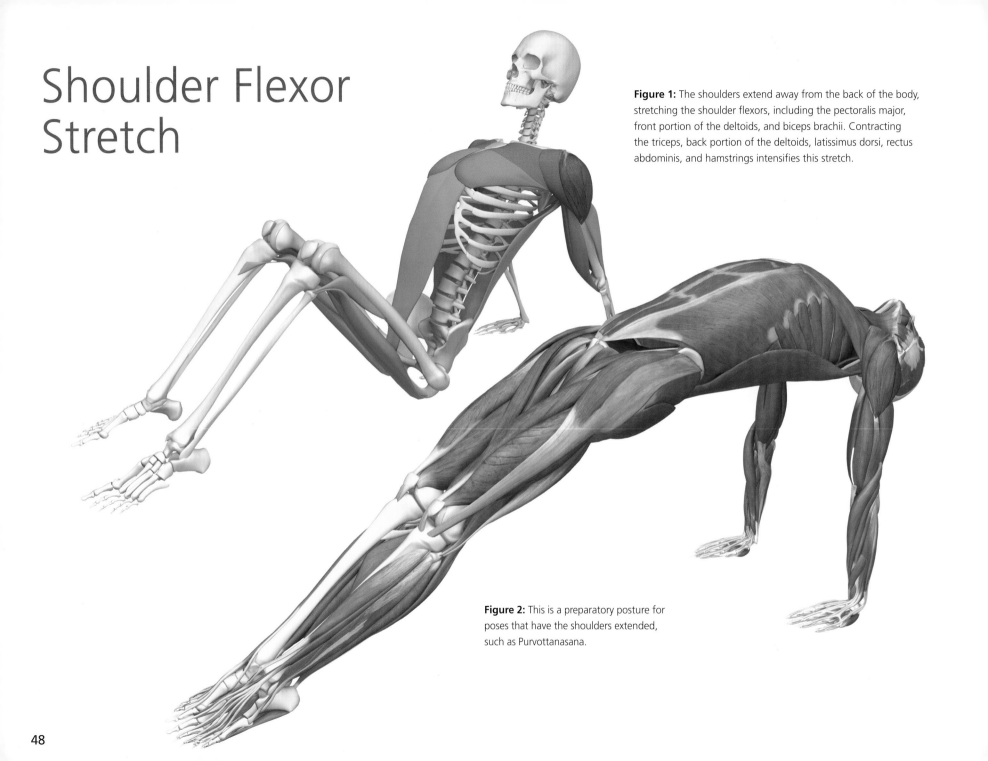

Figure 1: The shoulders extend away from the back of the body, stretching the shoulder flexors, including the pectoralis major, front portion of the deltoids, and biceps brachii. Contracting the triceps, back portion of the deltoids, latissimus dorsi, rectus abdominis, and hamstrings intensifies this stretch.

Figure 2: This is a preparatory posture for poses that have the shoulders extended, such as Purvottanasana.

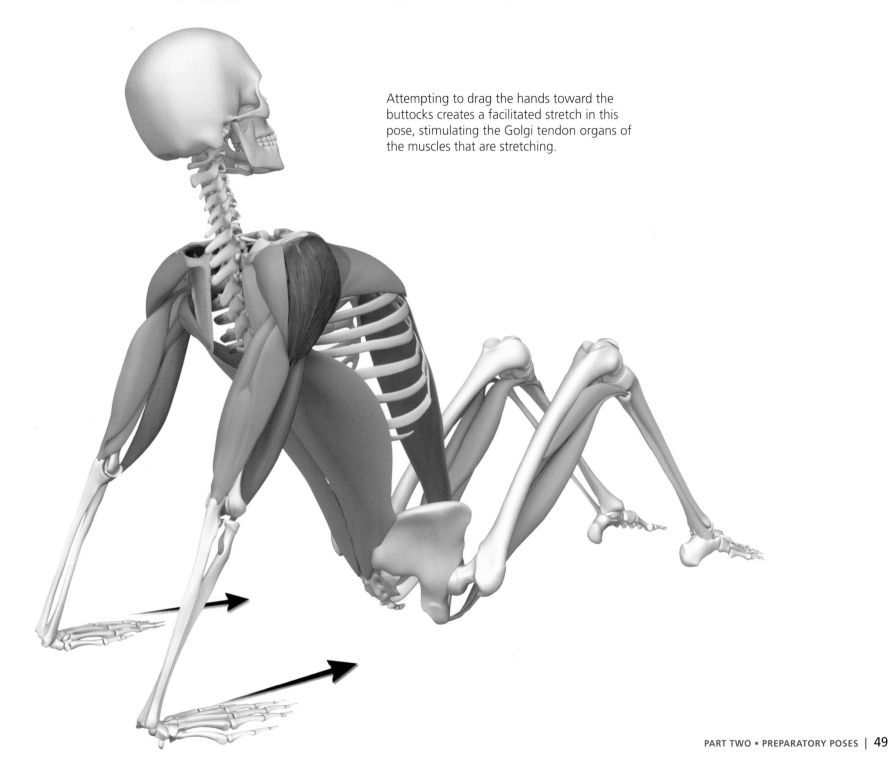

Attempting to drag the hands toward the buttocks creates a facilitated stretch in this pose, stimulating the Golgi tendon organs of the muscles that are stretching.

Surya Namaskar
Sun Salutations

The Sun Salutations are a combination of poses practiced in series, with each pose successively deepening with every repetition. It is typically performed at the start of the practice, classically upon awakening in the morning. In this way, the Sun Salutations can be viewed as a type of warm-up for the full practice.

Heat is generated in the body, raising the core temperature and causing the blood vessels on the body surface to dilate. Vasodilatation combines with sweating to dissipate the heat and regulate the core temperature of the body. Sweating also releases toxins from the body.

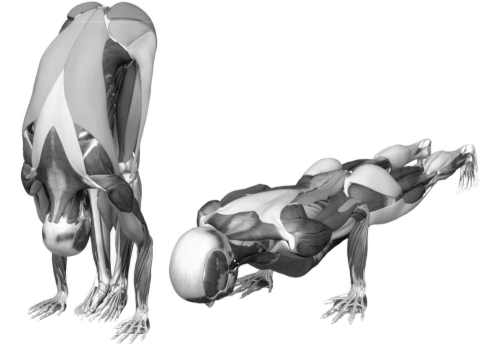

The increased heat raises blood flow to the muscles and makes the tendons and ligaments more pliable. Synovial fluid circulates in the joints, carrying nutrients to the articular cartilage and removing debris from the joint space.

The brain creates "set lengths" for muscles based on regular activity. Sitting in a chair or riding a bicycle on a regular basis signals the brain to set the length of the muscles about the hips for flexion. Consistent practice of Yoga lengthens the muscles, improving range of motion throughout the body. This creates new "set lengths" in the brain. Muscles tend to shorten when we sleep, accounting for "stiffness" in the morning. The Sun Salutations are a variation of ballistic stretching. Use this type of stretch to take the muscles back out to the length that was set in the brain during your previous practice.

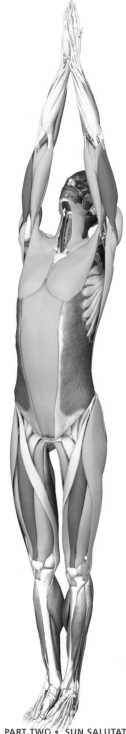
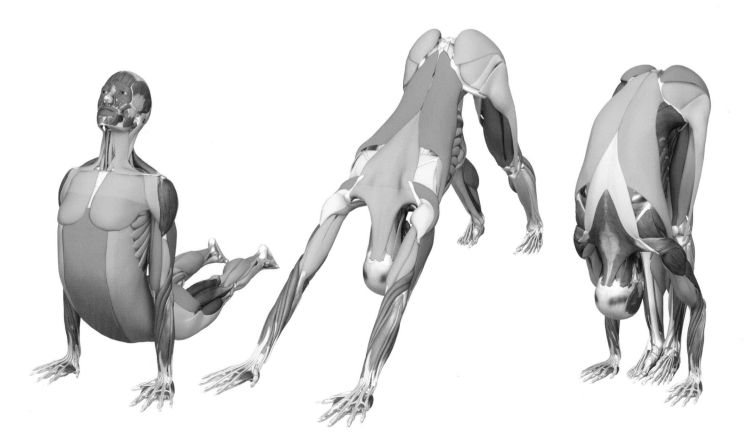

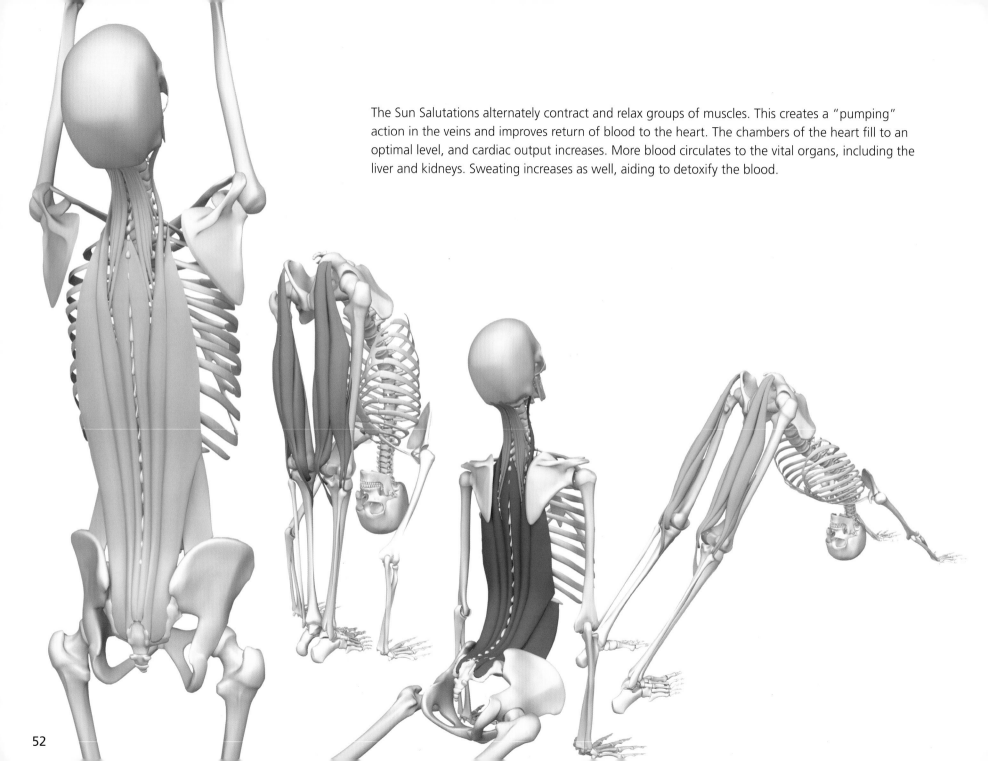

The Sun Salutations alternately contract and relax groups of muscles. This creates a "pumping" action in the veins and improves return of blood to the heart. The chambers of the heart fill to an optimal level, and cardiac output increases. More blood circulates to the vital organs, including the liver and kidneys. Sweating increases as well, aiding to detoxify the blood.

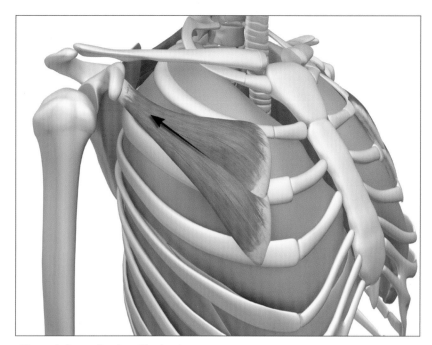

Figure 1: Pectoralis minor lifts the chest.

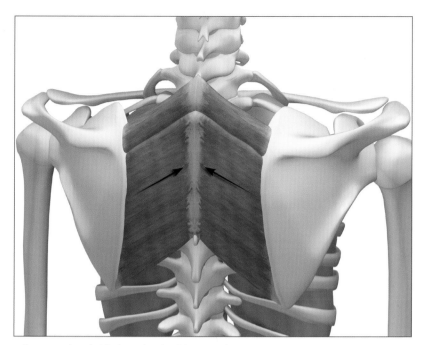

Figure 2: Rhomboids draw the shoulders together.

The Accessory Muscles of Breathing

Combining breath and body movement is a fundamental concept for practicing Yoga. The diaphragm and accessory breathing muscles move air in and out of the lungs. This action oxygenates the blood and removes carbon dioxide. The rate and depth of breathing also aids to regulate the pH of the tissues. Flow of the breath is regulated in the pharynx at the level of the glottis. Partial closure of the glottis increases air flow turbulence. This action brings more of the air into contact with the blood-rich mucosa of the nasal passages, warming the breath.

Breathing is among the most primitive of body functions. It is controlled and regulated by primal regions of the brain. We tap into these powerful regions of the brain by focusing on our breathing and combining breath with the movements of Yoga.

The images on this page illustrate how to open the rib cage using the accessory muscles of breathing. This technique is known as "bucket handle" breathing.

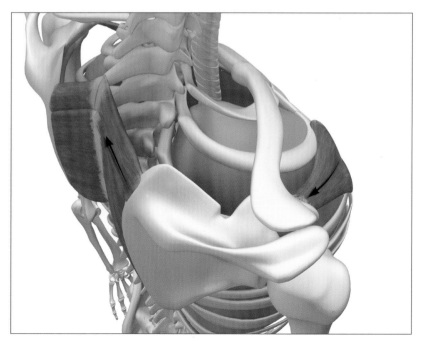

Figure 3: Pectoralis minor and rhomboids work in unison to open the chest.

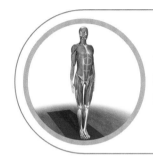

Tadasana
Mountain Pose
Page 56

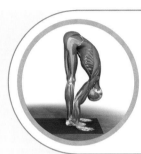

Uttanasana
Intense
Forward-Bending Pose
Page 58

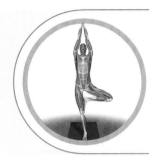

Vrksasana
Tree Pose
Page 60

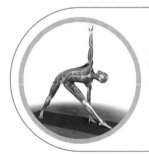

**Utthita
Trikonasana**
Extended Triangle Pose
Page 62

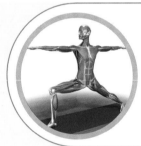

Virabhadrasana II
Warrior II
Page 64

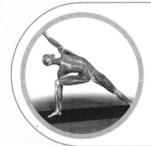

**Utthita
Parsvakonasana**
Extended Lateral
Angle Pose
Page 66

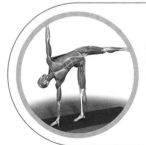

**Ardha
Chandrasana**
Half Moon Pose
Page 68

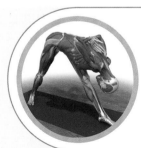

Parsvottanasana
Intense Side
Stretch Pose
Page 70

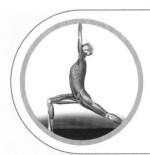

Virabhadrasana I
Warrior I
Page 72

Standing Poses

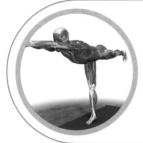

Virabhadrasana III
Warrior III
Page 74

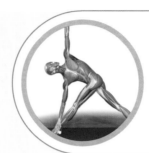

Parivrtta Trikonasana
Revolving Triangle Pose
Page 76

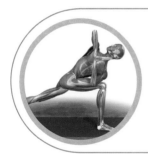

Parivrtta Parsvakonasana
Revolving Lateral Angle Pose
Page 78

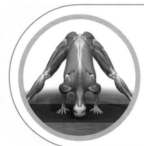

Prasarita Padottanasana
Spread Feet Intense Stretch Pose
Page 80

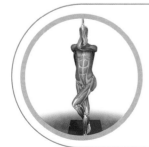

Garudasana
Eagle Pose
Page 82

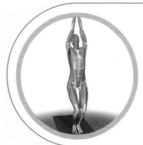

Utkatasana
Chair Pose
Page 84

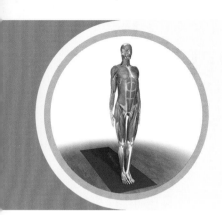

Tadasana: Mountain Pose

Tadasana precedes and follows the other standing poses. It is as though we have climbed to a plateau to gauge the transformative effects of our practice and collect our muscle-thoughts before continuing our ascent.

Synergizing/Activating

Pelvis and Legs

1. The muscles that keep the pelvis upright, like a bowl, are located front and back. At the front of the pelvis is the psoas, and at the back are the glutei or buttocks muscles. The pelvis is kept balanced because the psoas flexes the thigh, and the glutei make the thigh lengthen, or extend. These two muscles balance each other.

2. If the legs tend to turn outward, the tensor fascia lata and the front part of the gluteus medius muscles at the front and highest points of the hip bones work to turn them inward.

3. The quadriceps muscles down the front of the thighs shorten to straighten the knees.

4. The calf muscles are working quietly to balance the ankles on the feet, the bedrock of mountain pose.

5. All this time, the muscles on the top and bottom of the feet balance each other, grounding the pose.

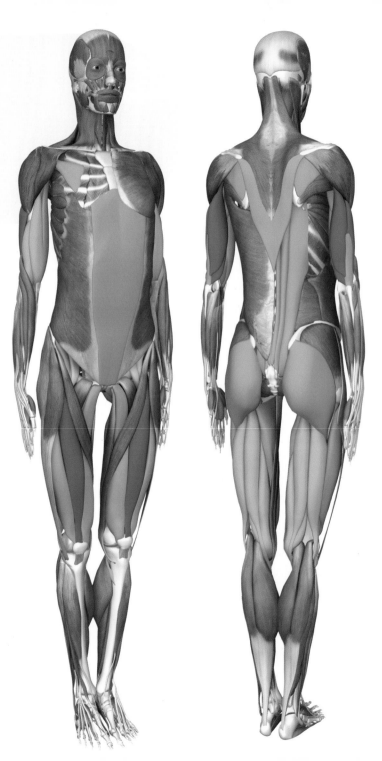

Trunk

1. The erector spinae (deeper back muscles) extend from the skull to the base of the spine and work with the muscles in the small of the back to lift the spine and hold you upright.

2. The abdominal muscles (running down the front of the trunk) work with the back muscles to support and balance the torso. Together they create a tube around the torso and draw the rib cage downward.

Shoulders and Arms

1. The lower part of the trapezius, which spans the back, draws the shoulders down and away from the ears, lifting the chest.

2. The muscles connecting the shoulder blades to the spinal column, the rhomboids, combine with the middle part of the trapezius to draw the shoulder blades toward the midline. This action opens the front of the chest.

3. The pectoralis minor muscle contracts in a closed-chain fashion to lift the lower ribs and open the chest.

4. Two muscles, the infraspinatus and teres minor, connect the shoulder blade to the upper arm bone and roll the arms outward.

5. The triceps straighten the elbows.

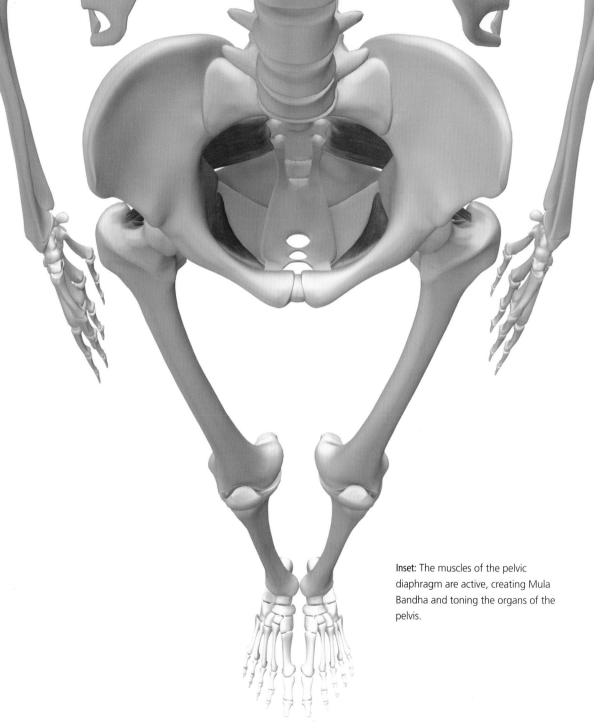

Inset: The muscles of the pelvic diaphragm are active, creating Mula Bandha and toning the organs of the pelvis.

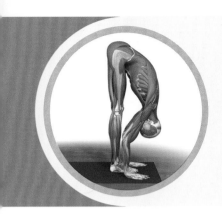

Uttanasana: Intense Forward-Bending Pose

Uttanasana is a symmetrical pose, offering the opportunity to identify asymmetry and imbalances between the two sides of the body. It is also a form of inversion, since it takes the head below the heart and is used during periods of rest in the practice.

Synergizing/Activating

Pelvis and Legs

1. The psoas, pectineus, and rectus femoris flex the hips and tilt the pelvis slightly forward.

2. The front part of the gluteus medius and the tensor fascia lata combine to turn the hips slightly inward so the kneecaps face directly forward.

3. The quadriceps, the large muscles down the front of the thighs, contract to straighten the knees. This action creates reciprocal inhibition, relaxing the muscles on the back of the thigh (the hamstrings).

4. The thighs are drawn together by the adductor muscles on the inside of each thigh.

Trunk, Shoulders, and Arms

1. The large band-like muscle on the front of the abdomen, the rectus abdominis, contracts to bend the trunk forward.

2. The lower part of the trapezius, which spans the back, draws the shoulders away from the neck.

3. The front part of the deltoids moves the shoulders forward. The biceps bend the elbows. When the hands are fixed on the ground, these actions push the trunk deeper into the pose.

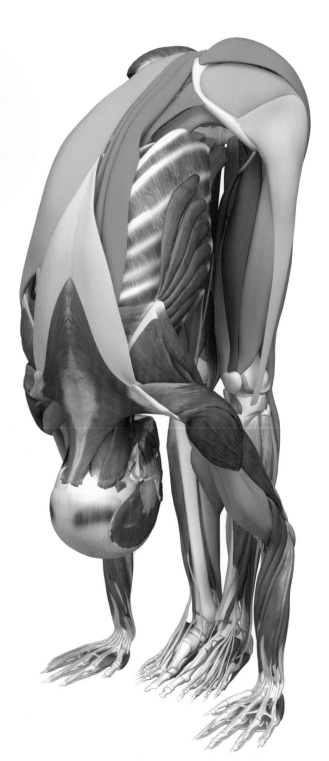

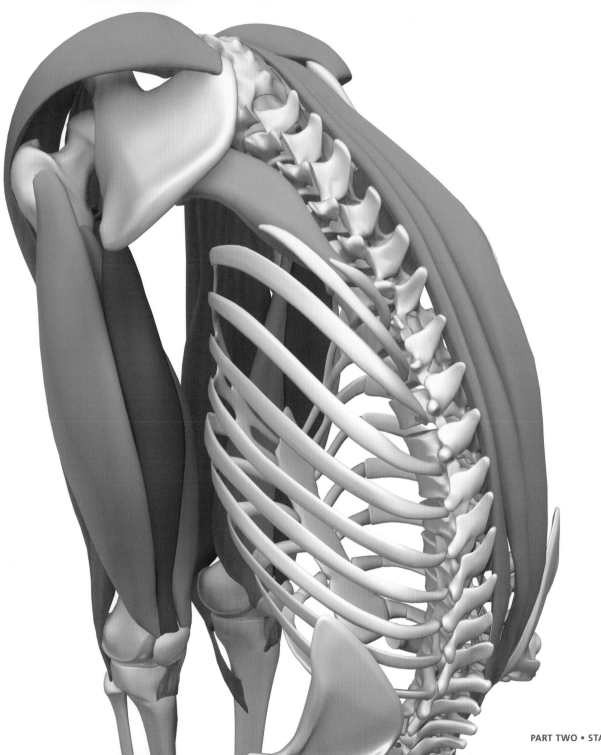
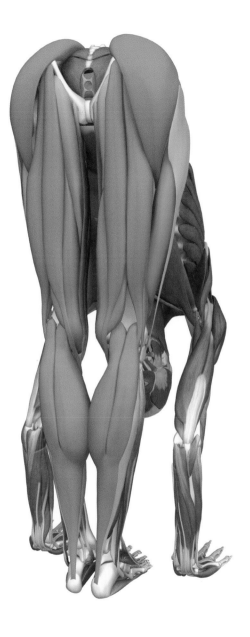

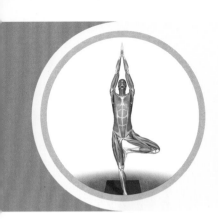

Vrksasana: Tree Pose

As the name suggests, this standing pose involves balancing on one leg with the arms together and reaching skyward, like a sapling. It is considered the easier of the one-legged balancing poses, because the bones of the upper body are stacked over the long bones of the standing leg. This leaves the trunk muscles and other muscle groups with less work when balancing the limbs.

Synergizing/Activating

Standing Leg

1. The gluteus maximus in the buttocks works with the psoas (located high at the front of the thigh) to balance the pelvis from front to back.

2. The gluteus medius on the outside of the pelvis and the adductor group on the inside of the thigh balance the pelvis from the outside to the inside.

3. The quadriceps down the front of the thigh shorten to straighten the knee.

4. The calf muscles, peronei and tibialis anterior, and toe flexors work in concert to stabilize the foot.

Trunk

1. The erector spinae, stretching from the skull to the backbone near the pelvis, hold the spine upright. They form a muscular column that works with the quadratus lumborum in the small of the back to lift the spine.

2. The rectus abdominis tethers the rib cage to the pelvis.

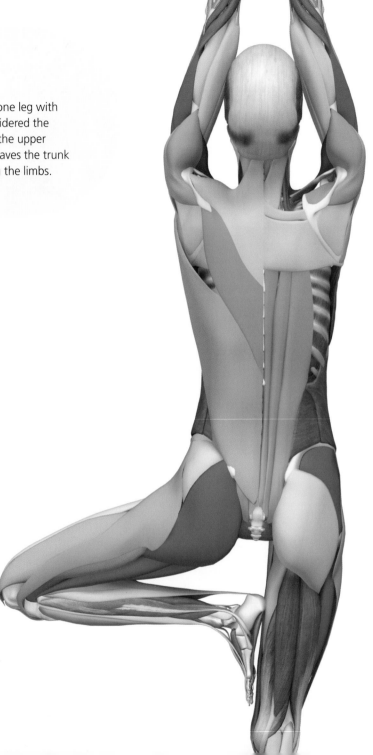

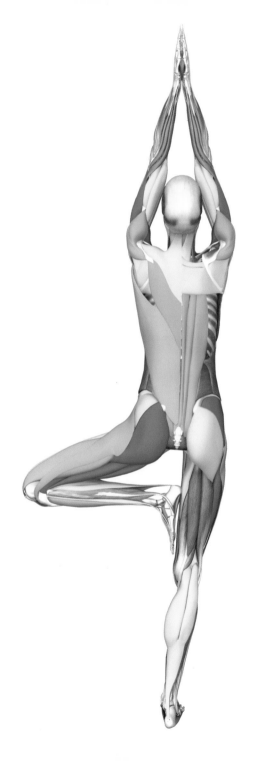

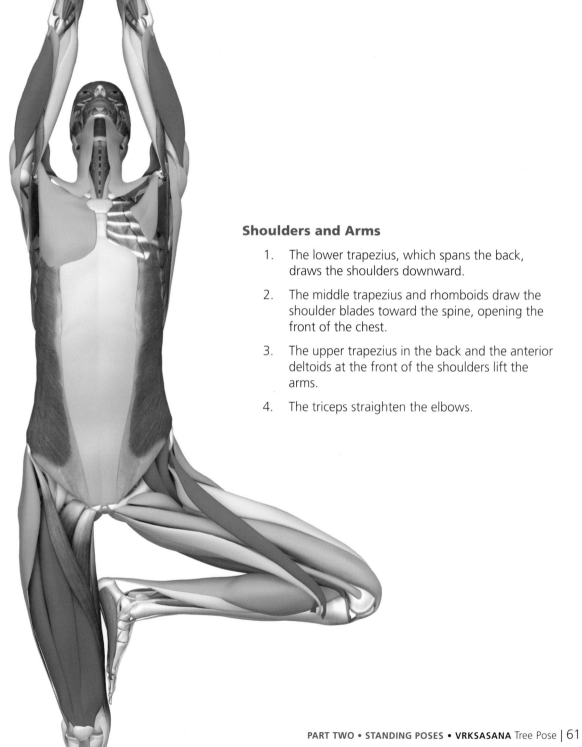

Shoulders and Arms

1. The lower trapezius, which spans the back, draws the shoulders downward.

2. The middle trapezius and rhomboids draw the shoulder blades toward the spine, opening the front of the chest.

3. The upper trapezius in the back and the anterior deltoids at the front of the shoulders lift the arms.

4. The triceps straighten the elbows.

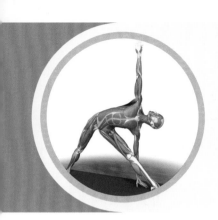

Utthita Trikonasana:
Extended Triangle Pose

Trikonasana creates a series of triangles with the body. These actions result in a powerful stretch of the front leg hamstrings, with a secondary stretch of the back leg hamstrings and gastroc-soleus muscles. It also stretches the upper-side abdominal and back muscles.

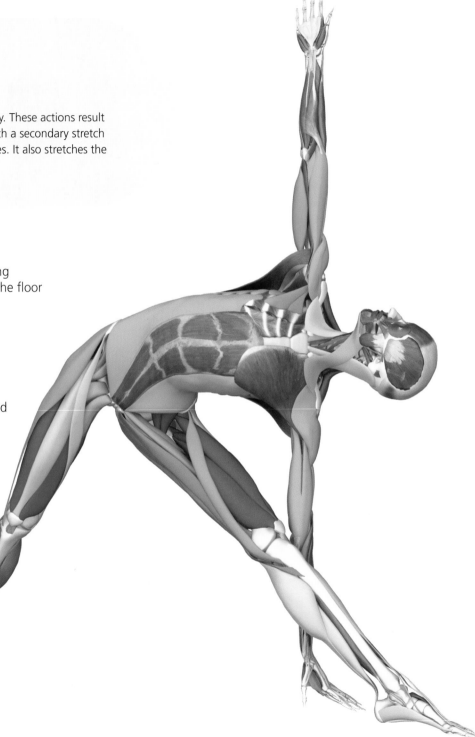

The upper side shoulder and upper arms have "open chain" movement, creating proprioceptive awareness of the arm in space. The lower side hand is fixed on the floor or leg, giving leverage to open the chest.

Synergizing/Activating

Pelvis and Legs

1. The front and back leg quadriceps contract, extending the knees and stretching the lower region of the hamstrings.

2. The front leg psoas flexes the hip and tilts the pelvis forward. This tilts the ischial tuberosity back, stretching the upper part of the front leg hamstrings.

3. The back leg gluteus maximus extends the hip.

4. The tibialis anterior of the back leg dorsiflexes the ankle, drawing it toward the shin.

5. The peroneus longus and brevis on the outside of the front shin activate, pressing the ball of the foot into the floor.

Trunk

1. The erector spinae, running along the length of the spine, are active, with the upper side turning the trunk slightly upward.

2. Muscles on the lower side of the abdomen, the obliques, activate to turn the torso upward. This action lengthens the obliques on the upper side of the trunk.

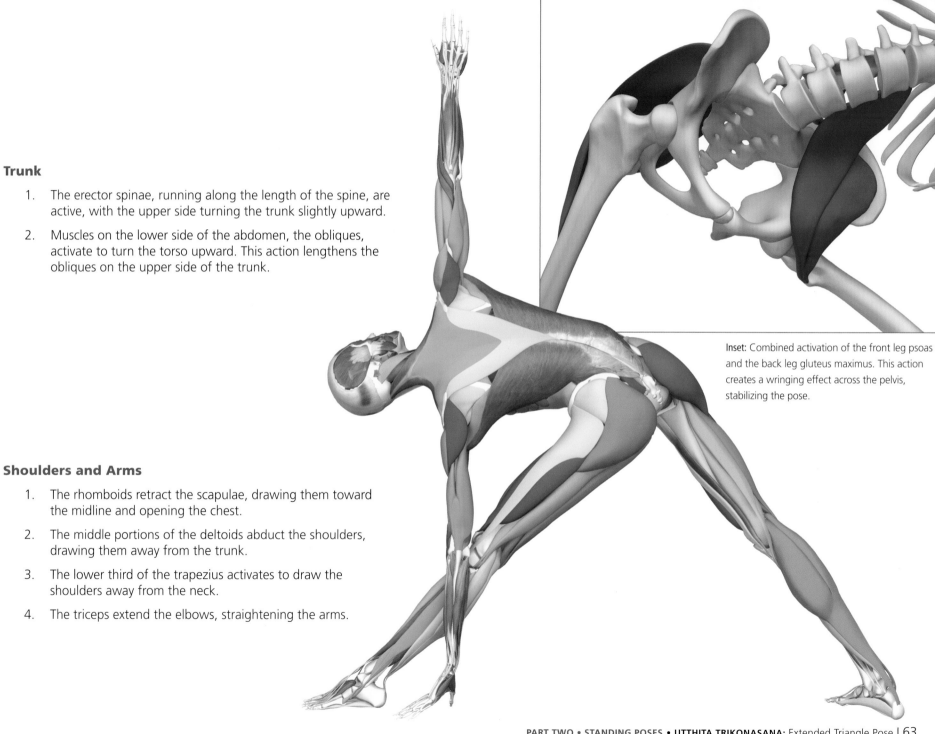

Inset: Combined activation of the front leg psoas and the back leg gluteus maximus. This action creates a wringing effect across the pelvis, stabilizing the pose.

Shoulders and Arms

1. The rhomboids retract the scapulae, drawing them toward the midline and opening the chest.

2. The middle portions of the deltoids abduct the shoulders, drawing them away from the trunk.

3. The lower third of the trapezius activates to draw the shoulders away from the neck.

4. The triceps extend the elbows, straightening the arms.

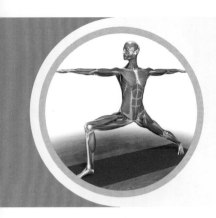

Virabhadrasana II: Warrior II

This version of the Warrior pose has the pelvis facing toward the front. Note that the progression of the standing poses in this book has the pelvis facing forward, then to the side, and finally turning. This sequence "walks" the effect of the poses around the core muscles of the pelvis, especially the psoas.

Synergizing/Activating

Pelvis and Legs

1. The back-leg buttock muscles extend and externally rotate the hip.

2. The back-leg adductor magnus extends the thigh bone and helps stabilize the foot on the floor.

3. The tensor fascia lata and gluteus medius turn the thigh bone inward, balancing the external rotation of the gluteus maximus.

4. The quadriceps straighten the back knee.

5. The muscle along the front of the shin, the tibialis anterior, bends the back ankle upward, stretching the calf muscles and those along the outside of the calf.

6. The muscle high on the front of the front hip, the pectineus, works with the psoas to bend the hip. A muscle mid-thigh, the sartorius, works to refine this action.

7. The front leg quadriceps contract to support the body weight.

8. Muscles along the outside of the front leg calf, the peronei, turn the ankle slightly outward, everting it. The net effect of this action presses the ball of the foot down.

9. The gastrocnemius and soleus press the sole of the foot into the floor.

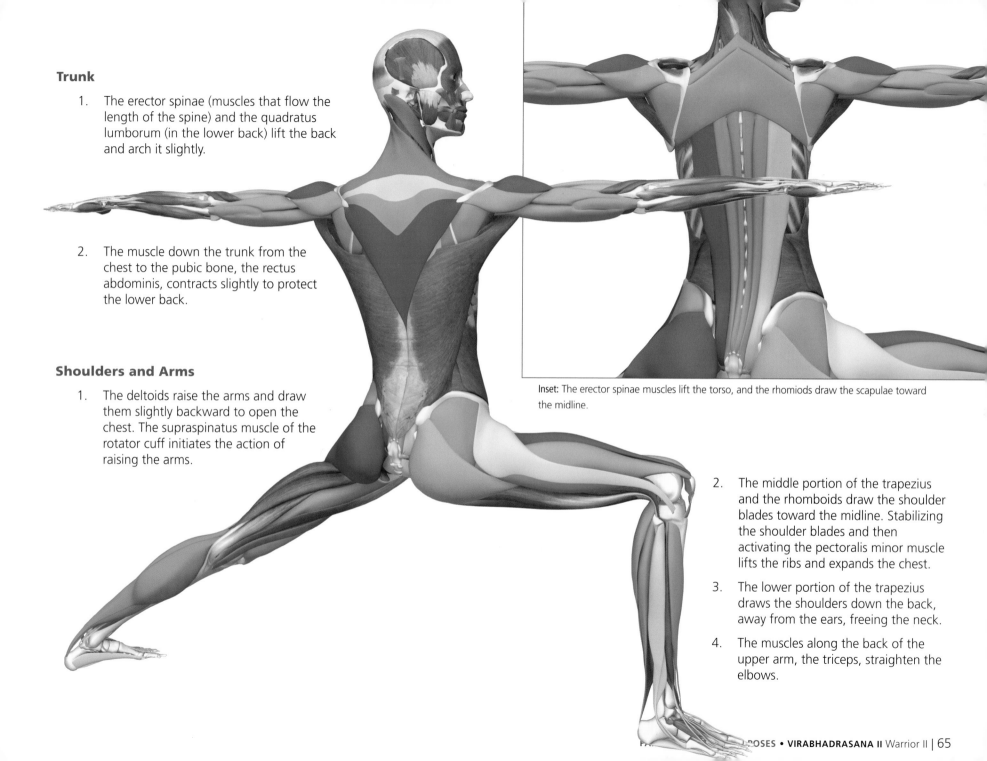

Trunk

1. The erector spinae (muscles that flow the length of the spine) and the quadratus lumborum (in the lower back) lift the back and arch it slightly.

2. The muscle down the trunk from the chest to the pubic bone, the rectus abdominis, contracts slightly to protect the lower back.

Shoulders and Arms

1. The deltoids raise the arms and draw them slightly backward to open the chest. The supraspinatus muscle of the rotator cuff initiates the action of raising the arms.

Inset: The erector spinae muscles lift the torso, and the rhomiods draw the scapulae toward the midline.

2. The middle portion of the trapezius and the rhomboids draw the shoulder blades toward the midline. Stabilizing the shoulder blades and then activating the pectoralis minor muscle lifts the ribs and expands the chest.

3. The lower portion of the trapezius draws the shoulders down the back, away from the ears, freeing the neck.

4. The muscles along the back of the upper arm, the triceps, straighten the elbows.

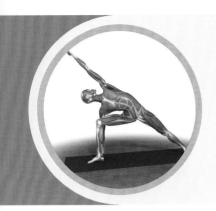

Utthita Parsvakonasana:
Extended Lateral Angle Pose

This is one of the standing poses in which the pelvis faces forward, parallel to the front plane of the body. It is the natural progression from Warrior II, with one hand placed on the floor and the other stretching upward over the head.

Synergizing/Activating

Pelvis and Legs

1. The back-leg buttock muscle extends the hip and turns it outward.

2. The adductor group of muscles on the inside of the thigh extend the femur and draw the leg toward the midline, stabilizing the back foot on the floor.

3. The tensor fascia lata and gluteus medius turn the hip inward. This balances the strong outward pull by the large buttock muscle.

4. The quadriceps, the muscles along the front of the thigh, straighten the back knee.

5. The muscle along the front of the shin, the tibialis anterior, draws the ankle toward the shin, which stretches the calf muscles and the muscles along the outside of the calf, the peroneus longus and brevis.

6. The psoas and pectineus muscles bend the hip of the front leg. The muscle crossing diagonally over the midline of the thigh, the sartorius, refines this action.

7. The quadriceps of the front leg activates to support the body weight.

8. The peroneus muscles along the outside of the front leg calf turn the ankle slightly outward, everting it. The gastrocnemius/soleus presses the foot into the floor by flexing the ankle.

Trunk

1. The lower-side abdominal oblique and transverse muscle draws the trunk toward the bent leg, stretching the same muscles on the upper side of the trunk.

2. On the lower side, the muscles along the spine and those in the lower back (the erector spinae and quadratus lumborum) bend the trunk to the side, stretching the corresponding muscles on the upper side.

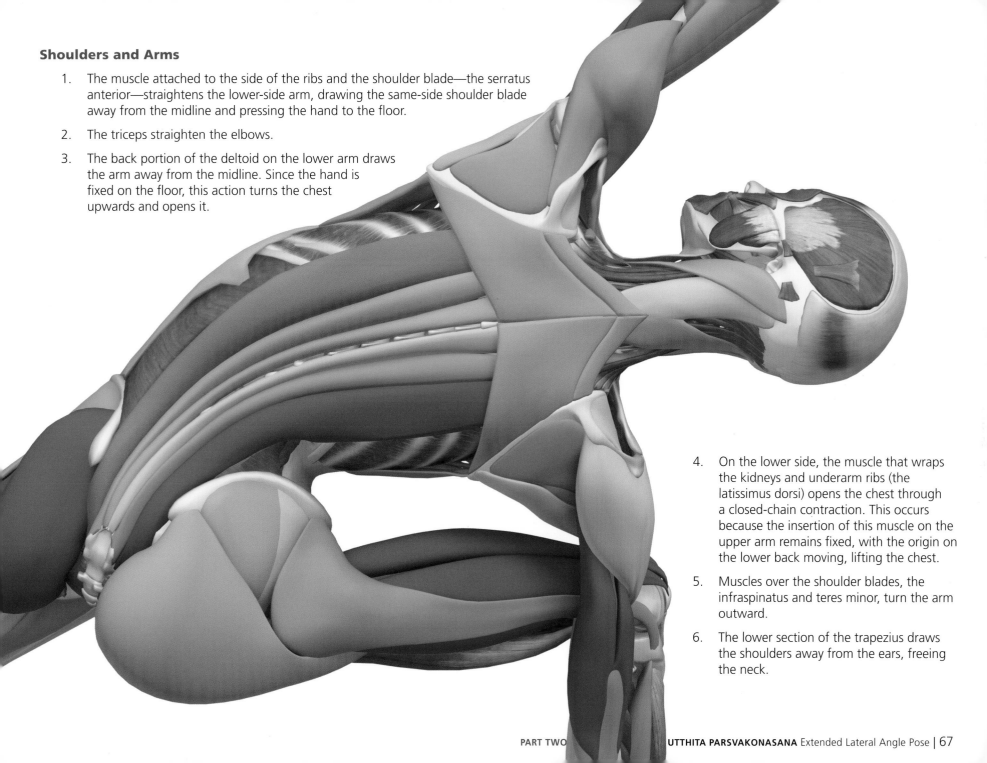

Shoulders and Arms

1. The muscle attached to the side of the ribs and the shoulder blade—the serratus anterior—straightens the lower-side arm, drawing the same-side shoulder blade away from the midline and pressing the hand to the floor.

2. The triceps straighten the elbows.

3. The back portion of the deltoid on the lower arm draws the arm away from the midline. Since the hand is fixed on the floor, this action turns the chest upwards and opens it.

4. On the lower side, the muscle that wraps the kidneys and underarm ribs (the latissimus dorsi) opens the chest through a closed-chain contraction. This occurs because the insertion of this muscle on the upper arm remains fixed, with the origin on the lower back moving, lifting the chest.

5. Muscles over the shoulder blades, the infraspinatus and teres minor, turn the arm outward.

6. The lower section of the trapezius draws the shoulders away from the ears, freeing the neck.

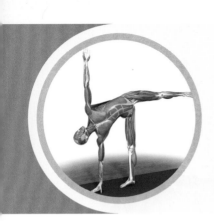

Ardha Chandrasana: Half Moon Pose

In this pose, the body weight is on one leg, with one hand extended and touching the floor. The other leg is extended parallel to the floor and acts as an active counterbalance. Freely interpreted, the pose carves a half moon; ideally, it hangs quietly in the sky. All limbs must remain on the same plane, because tipping the leg backwards will cause loss of balance. The Half Moon requires some knowledge of the core pelvic muscles and how to engage them so the leg can move freely.

Synergizing/Activating

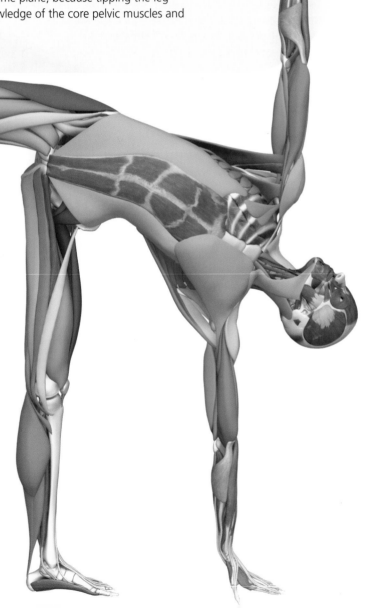

Standing Leg

1. The psoas and pectineus tilt the hip slightly forward. One of the muscles that crosses the hip and runs down the front of the thigh—the rectus femoris—works in concert with the other two muscles to stabilize the leg. The sartorius, a muscle that runs down the front of the thigh at an angle, further stabilizes the pose.

2. The quadriceps straighten the knee.

3. The calf muscles, the gastrocnemius and soleus, eccentrically contract to press the foot down, grounding the pose.

Lifting Leg

1. The muscles originating from the side of the pelvis, gluteus medius, gluteus minimus, and tensor fascia lata, lift the leg parallel to the floor.

2. The gluteus maximus in the buttocks works with the psoas high at the front of the thigh to keep the hip from swaying front to back.

3. The quadriceps straighten the knee.

4. The tibialis anterior and peronei muscles along the shin and the calf engage to stabilize the foot.

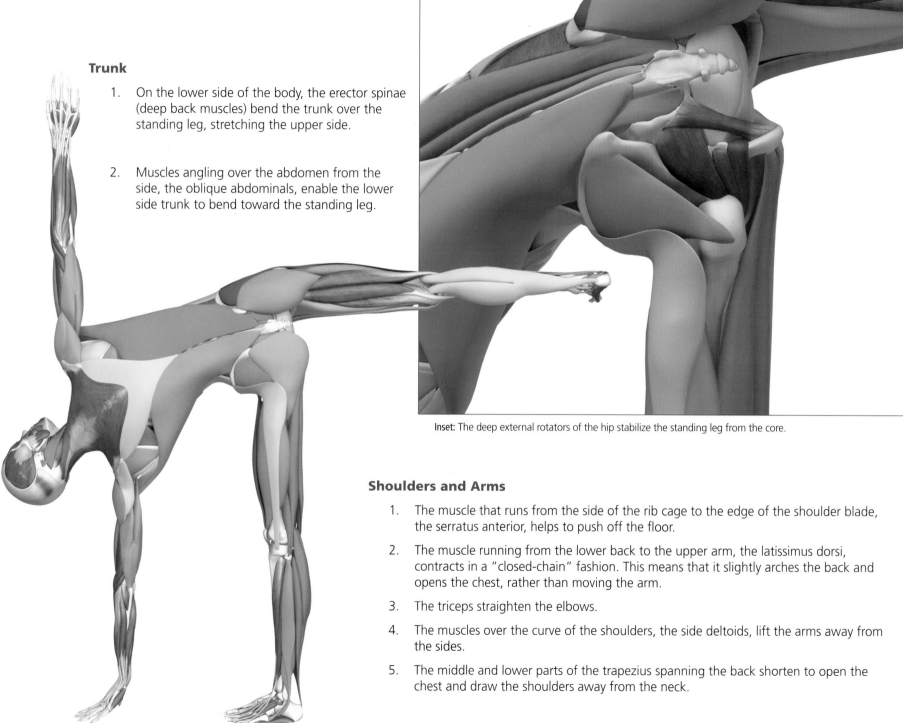

Trunk

1. On the lower side of the body, the erector spinae (deep back muscles) bend the trunk over the standing leg, stretching the upper side.

2. Muscles angling over the abdomen from the side, the oblique abdominals, enable the lower side trunk to bend toward the standing leg.

Inset: The deep external rotators of the hip stabilize the standing leg from the core.

Shoulders and Arms

1. The muscle that runs from the side of the rib cage to the edge of the shoulder blade, the serratus anterior, helps to push off the floor.

2. The muscle running from the lower back to the upper arm, the latissimus dorsi, contracts in a "closed-chain" fashion. This means that it slightly arches the back and opens the chest, rather than moving the arm.

3. The triceps straighten the elbows.

4. The muscles over the curve of the shoulders, the side deltoids, lift the arms away from the sides.

5. The middle and lower parts of the trapezius spanning the back shorten to open the chest and draw the shoulders away from the neck.

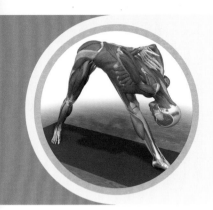

Parsvottanasana: Intense Side Stretch Pose

Parsvottanasana intensely stretches the muscles at the back of the thighs and two muscles in the calf of the back leg, the gastrocnemius and the soleus. Placing the hands in Namasté behind the back rotates the shoulders inward and intensely stretches the muscles that turn the bone in the upper arm outward, the infraspinatus and teres minor.

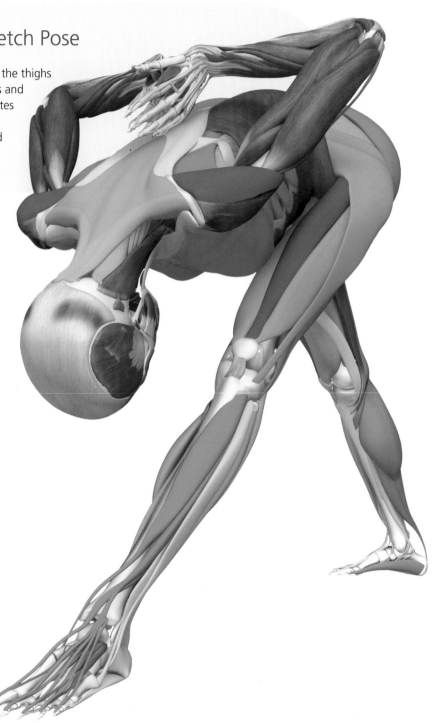

Synergizing/Activating

1. The pectoralis major works with the subscapularis and teres major to turn the upper arm bone inward and stretch the external rotators of the shoulder, the infraspinatus and teres minor.

2. Muscles spanning the upper back, the middle trapezius and rhomboids, pull the shoulder blades toward the spine to open the front of the chest.

3. The lower trapezius draws the shoulders down the back, freeing the neck.

4. The rectus abdominis bends the trunk toward the thigh.

5. The psoas works two ways: it helps the front hip bend and it holds the back hip steady, stabilizing the extended leg.

6. The buttocks muscles extend the thigh bone of the back leg. The back foot is fixed on the mat. Thus the energy from extending the thigh bone is felt at the back of the knee, increasing the stretch of the hamstrings and the calf muscles down the length of the back leg.

7. The quadriceps of both legs straighten the knees.

8. The muscle beside the shin of the back leg, the tibialis anterior, shortens to allow that ankle to bend toward the shin, enabling the calf muscles to stretch more.

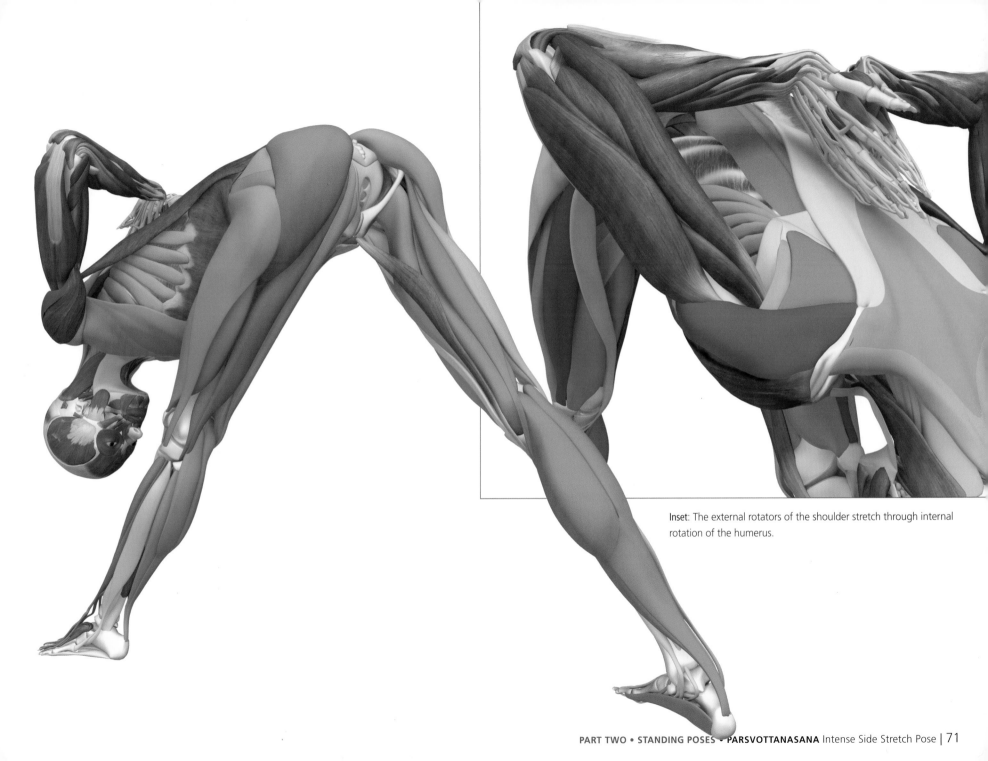

Inset: The external rotators of the shoulder stretch through internal rotation of the humerus.

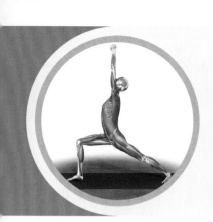

Virabhadrasana I: Warrior I

This fundamental standing pose is a type of lunge with the torso extending and the chest opening upward. Although a still posture, Warrior I suggests disciplined muscle energy waiting to be unleashed.

Synergizing/Activating

Pelvis and Legs

1. The buttock muscle of the back leg extends and turns the hip outward.

2. The tensor fascia lata works with the gluteus medius to move the femur away from the center line (abduction). At the same time, they offset the action of the buttock muscle, turning the hip outward in its socket by rotating the thigh bone inward.

3. The large muscle along the inside of the thigh, the adductor magnus, extends and moves the thigh bone toward the center line.

4. The quadriceps straighten the knee.

5. The muscle along the front of the shin, the tibialis anterior, shortens to allow the ankle to bend and stretches the back leg calf muscles, as well as those along the outside of the shin, the peroneus longus and brevis.

6. At the same time, the front leg bends at the hip, aided by the shortening of the psoas and pectineus. Balance is assisted by the sartorius bending the hip and turning the thigh outward.

7. The front leg quadriceps muscles contract to support the body weight.

8. Muscles along the outer aspect of the shin, the peroneus longus and brevis, turn the ankle and the front foot slightly outward, pressing the ball of the foot into the floor.

9. The calf muscle presses the sole of the foot into the floor.

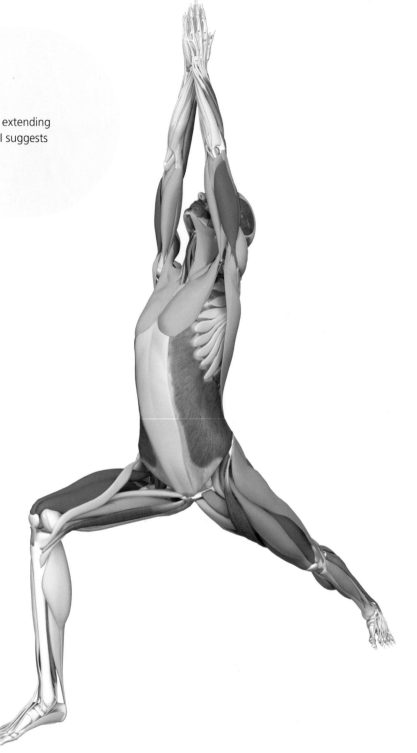

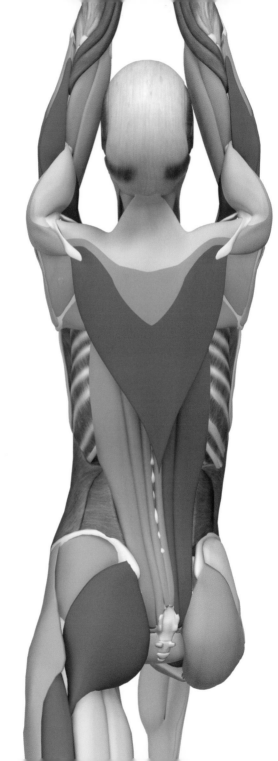

Trunk

1. The erector spinae muscles, stretching from the skull down to the backbone near the pelvis, work with the quadratus lumborum muscle in the lumbar spine to lift the back and arch it slightly.

2. The rectus abdominis is engaged to contract slightly, helping protect the lower back.

Shoulders and Arms

1. The lower part of the trapezius muscle, which spans the back, draws the shoulders down the back, freeing the neck.

2. The muscles running from the side of the rib cage to the shoulder blade, the serratus anterior, turn the lower edge of the shoulder blade outward. This action moves the socket part of the shoulder joint under the head of the humerus (in the shoulder joint).

3. The infraspinatus and teres minor roll the arm bones outward, opening the chest.

4. The front part of the deltoids activates and shortens to raise the arms.

5. The triceps straighten the elbows, while assisting the serratus anterior in rotating the scapulae. This action prevents impingement of the humeral head on the acromion process of the scapula.

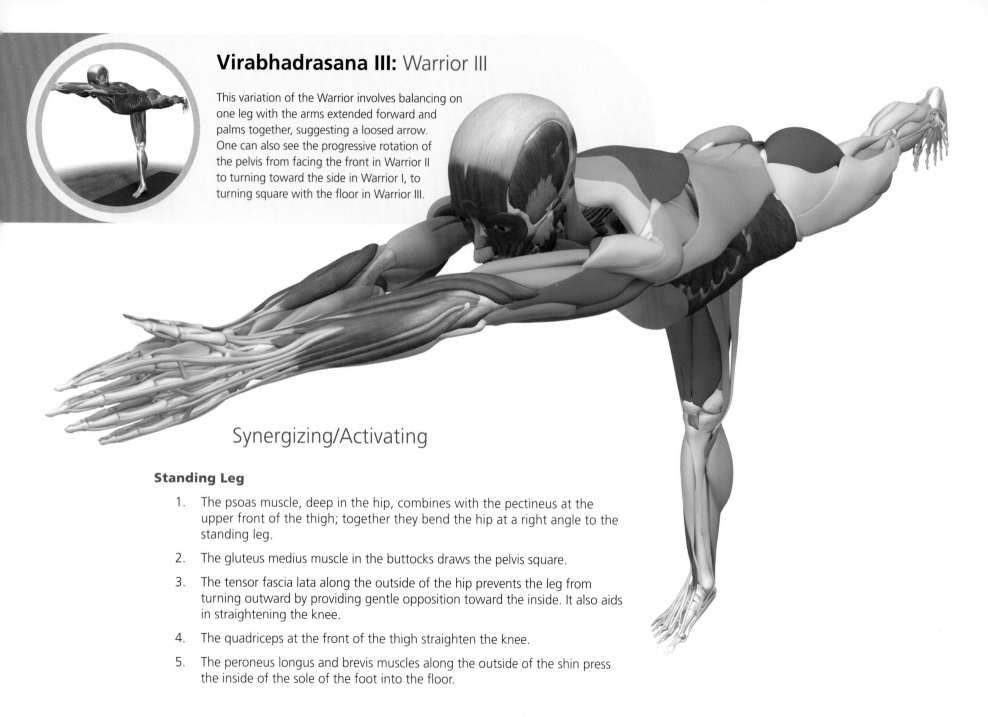

Virabhadrasana III: Warrior III

This variation of the Warrior involves balancing on one leg with the arms extended forward and palms together, suggesting a loosed arrow. One can also see the progressive rotation of the pelvis from facing the front in Warrior II to turning toward the side in Warrior I, to turning square with the floor in Warrior III.

Synergizing/Activating

Standing Leg

1. The psoas muscle, deep in the hip, combines with the pectineus at the upper front of the thigh; together they bend the hip at a right angle to the standing leg.

2. The gluteus medius muscle in the buttocks draws the pelvis square.

3. The tensor fascia lata along the outside of the hip prevents the leg from turning outward by providing gentle opposition toward the inside. It also aids in straightening the knee.

4. The quadriceps at the front of the thigh straighten the knee.

5. The peroneus longus and brevis muscles along the outside of the shin press the inside of the sole of the foot into the floor.

Lifting Leg

1. The gluteus maximus and posterior fibers of the gluteus medius lift the leg.

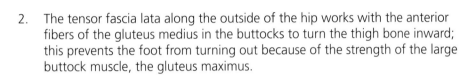

2. The tensor fascia lata along the outside of the hip works with the anterior fibers of the gluteus medius in the buttocks to turn the thigh bone inward; this prevents the foot from turning out because of the strength of the large buttock muscle, the gluteus maximus.

3. The erector spinae cooperate with the quadratus lumborum in the small of the back to lift the pelvis.

4. The quadriceps along the front of the thigh straighten the knee.

5. The gastrocnemius/soleus calf muscles and the tibialis anterior and peronei on either side of the shin work in concert to stabilize the ankle and foot.

Trunk

1. The erector spinae back muscles and quadratus lumborum in the small of the back lift the spine. The rectus abdominis, running from the chest down to the pubic bone, creates a sheath around the torso to stabilize it.

Shoulders and Arms

1. The upper trapezius spanning the back draws the shoulder blades toward the midline and down the back. It also aids in lifting the arms.

2. The infraspinatus and teres minor muscles connecting the shoulder blade to the upper arm bone, the humerus, turn that bone outward. This prevents the arm bone from coming into contact with the acromion, a bony structure on the scapula that forms a joint with the collarbone.

3. The anterior deltoids over the front of the shoulder lift the arms.

4. The triceps straighten the elbows.

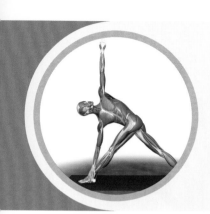

Parivrtta Trikonasana: Revolving Triangle Pose

The Revolving Triangle is a pose that connects the opposite-side hand to the foot, transmitting a twist across the trunk and spine. The core muscles of the shoulder turn the trunk in the opposite direction of the hips, creating the twist.

Synergizing/Activating

1. The front leg psoas conspires with the back leg buttock muscles to create a wringing effect across the pelvis, thus stabilizing the pose.

2. The same psoas works with the pectineus, a muscle connecting the thigh bone to the pubic bone, and the adductor muscles to bend the front-leg hip.

3. Meanwhile, the back-leg buttock muscle extends the leg behind the body and turns it outward.

4. The large inner thigh muscle of the back leg, the adductor magnus, presses that thigh bone back and draws it toward the center line.

5. The quadriceps straighten the knees.

6. In the back leg, the muscle along the edge of the shin (the tibialis anterior) turns the ankle slightly inward, drawing the top of the foot toward the shin. This action stretches the muscles in the back of the calf.

7. The triceps straighten the elbows.

8. A muscle at the side of the rib cage and connected to the shoulder blade, the serratus anterior, draws the lower arm shoulder down to the foot.

9. The back portion of the lower arm deltoid persuades the trunk to turn farther into the twist by drawing the chest forward.

10. Muscles connecting the shoulder blade to the spine (the rhomboids) and the back portion of the deltoid draw the upper side of the trunk deeper into the twist.

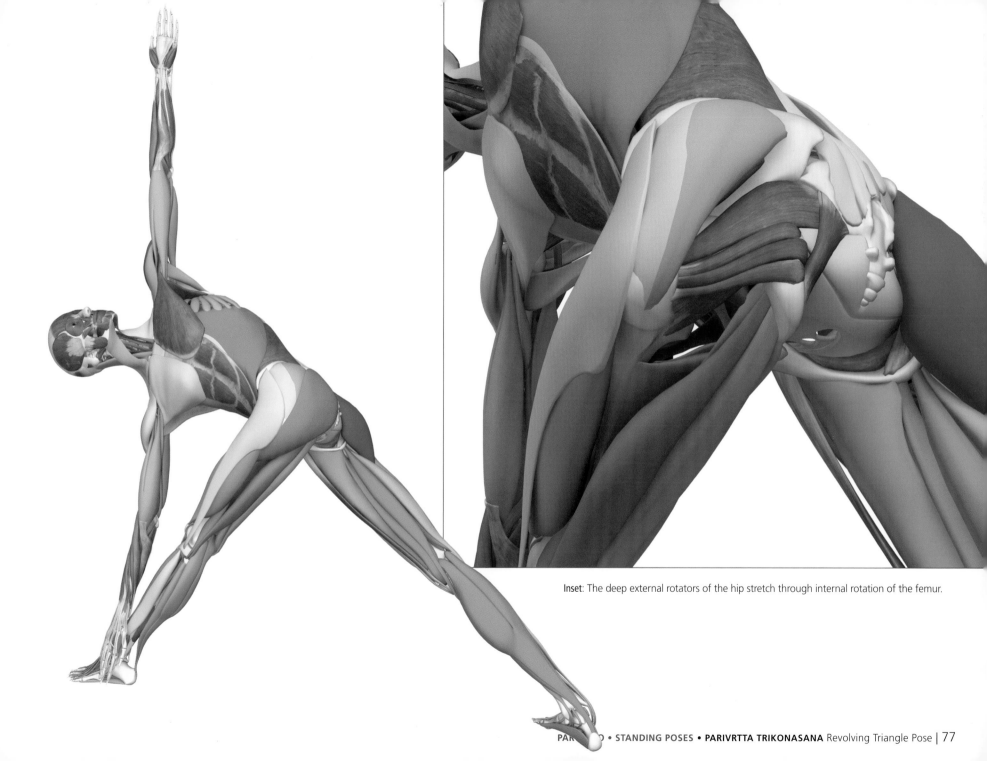

Inset: The deep external rotators of the hip stretch through internal rotation of the femur.

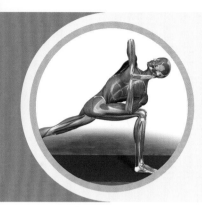

Parivrtta Parsvakonasana:
Revolving Lateral Angle Pose (Lunge Variation)

Parivrtta Parsvakonasana turns the pelvis and trunk in opposite directions. This action creates a stretch of the core muscles surrounding the spine. Stabilize this pose by activating the front leg psoas and back leg gluteus maximus. The result is a "wringing" effect across the pelvis, where there is pull and counter-pull from the muscles, ligaments, and tendons around the pelvis. Pushing off with the back foot and resisting with the front foot further stabilizes the pose.

Synergizing/Activating

1. The muscles on the inside and front of the front hip/thigh work together to bend that hip. These are the psoas, pectineus, and anterior adductors.

2. Muscles along the outside of the front hip and those beside the large buttock muscle cooperate to press the knee against the elbow, aiding in the turn of the pose. These are the tensor fascia lata and gluteus medius.

3. The muscles along the outside of the lower leg, the peronei, help press the ball of the front foot downward and turn the ankle slightly outward, everting it.

4. The large buttock muscle, the gluteus maximus, moves the back hip to the rear and turns it outward.

5. The back hip is pressed farther back and also drawn toward the midline by the large muscle along the inside of the thigh, the adductor magnus.

6. The quadriceps straighten the back knee.

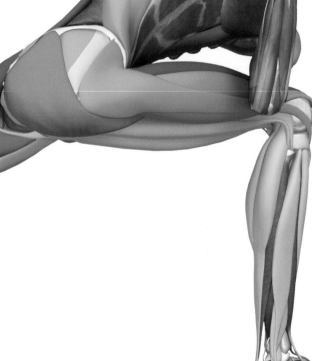

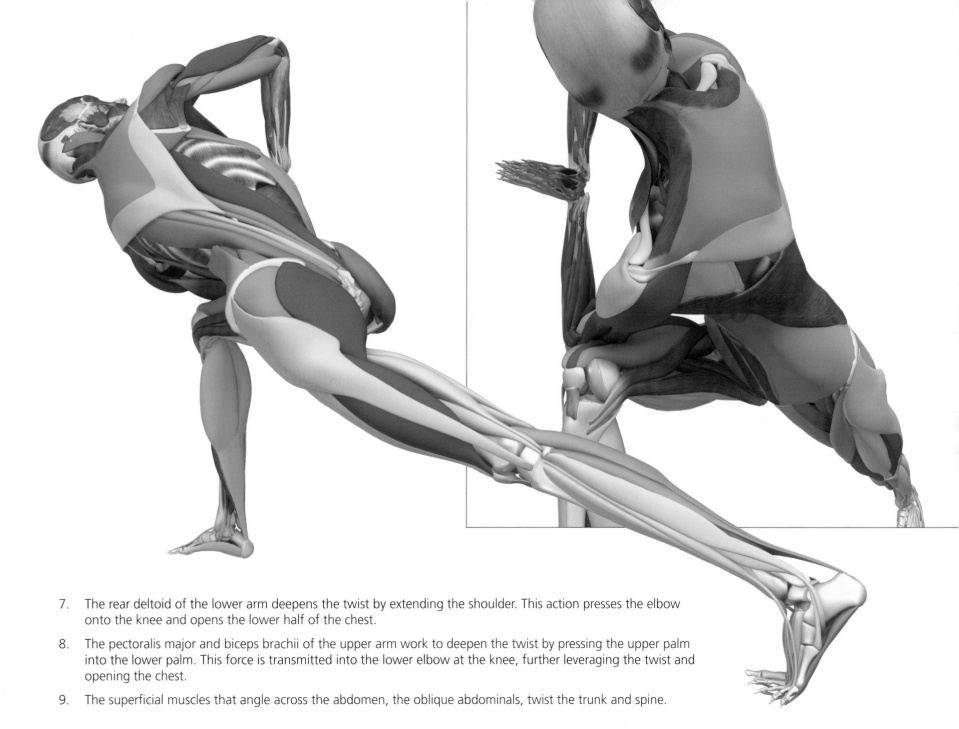

7. The rear deltoid of the lower arm deepens the twist by extending the shoulder. This action presses the elbow onto the knee and opens the lower half of the chest.

8. The pectoralis major and biceps brachii of the upper arm work to deepen the twist by pressing the upper palm into the lower palm. This force is transmitted into the lower elbow at the knee, further leveraging the twist and opening the chest.

9. The superficial muscles that angle across the abdomen, the oblique abdominals, twist the trunk and spine.

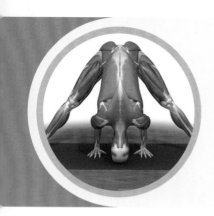

Prasarita Padottanasana: Spread Feet Intense Stretch Pose

Prasarita Padottanasana is a symmetrical standing pose in that both sides of the body are activated and stretched equally. This type of pose shows you the areas of the body that are not equal in flexibility. Once these areas are identified, activate the appropriate muscles to work toward symmetry.

Synergizing/Activating

1. The hips are bent by the psoas, pectineus, and rectus femoris muscles at the front of the thigh.

2. The quadriceps muscles along the front of the thighs straighten the knees.

3. The tibialis anterior muscles along the front of the shin turn the feet in slightly.

4. The tibialis posterior muscles, running on the inside of the ankles, help lift the arches.

5. The muscles along the bottom of the feet at the great toes, the flexor hallucis longii, press the fleshy part of the toe against the floor to aid in stability and draw the weight forward.

6. The rectus abdominis muscle, flowing from the chest to the pubic bone, bends the trunk forward.

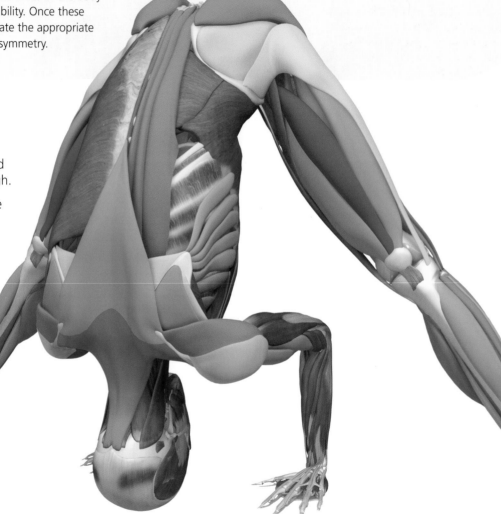

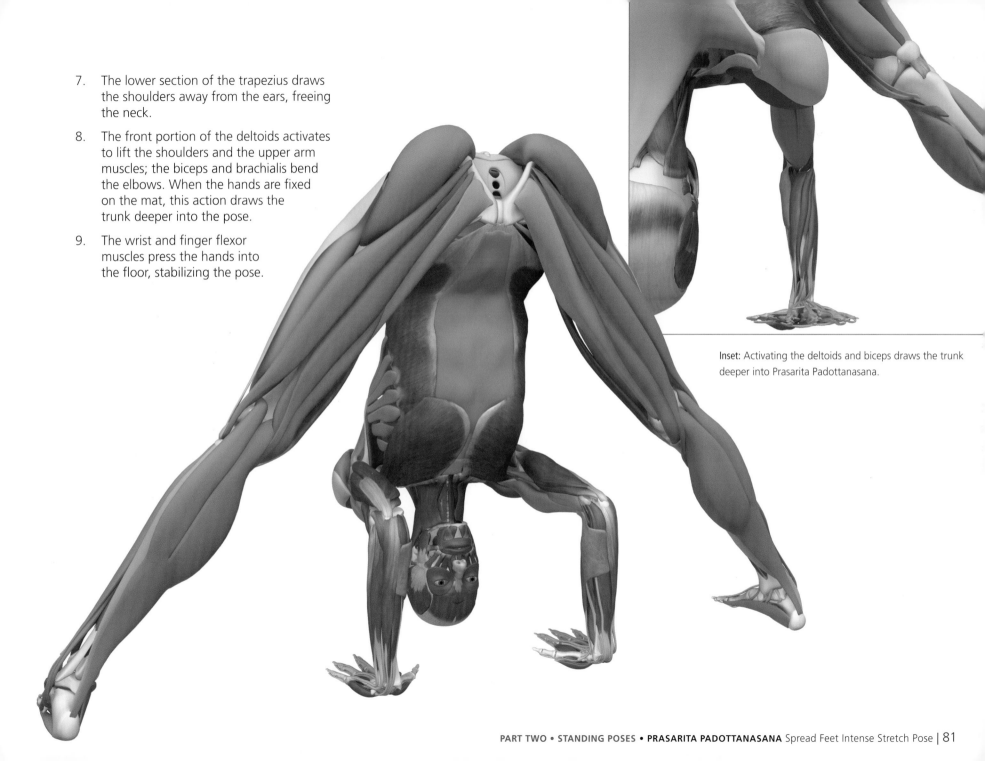

7. The lower section of the trapezius draws the shoulders away from the ears, freeing the neck.

8. The front portion of the deltoids activates to lift the shoulders and the upper arm muscles; the biceps and brachialis bend the elbows. When the hands are fixed on the mat, this action draws the trunk deeper into the pose.

9. The wrist and finger flexor muscles press the hands into the floor, stabilizing the pose.

Inset: Activating the deltoids and biceps draws the trunk deeper into Prasarita Padottanasana.

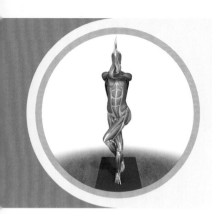

Garudasana: Eagle Pose

This pose involves balancing on one leg while the arms and legs are wrapped in a position not normally seen by the brain. As such, it is effective for training in balance and coordination.

Synergizing/Activating

Pelvis and Legs

1. The standing leg peronei evert the ankle to press the inside of the foot down, aiding in balancing.

2. The wrapping leg peronei evert the ankle to create a hook around the lower standing leg.

3. The gastrocnemius/soleus of the calf flexes the standing leg ankle to press the foot down, stabilizing the pose.

4. The adductor group squeezes the thighs together.

5. The tensor fascia lata and gluteus medius rotate the femurs internally.

6. The psoas flexes the hips.

Trunk

1. The erector spinae and quadratus lumborum lift the back.

2. The rectus abdominis provides a counterforce to the erector spinae, stabilizing the pelvis.

Shoulders and Arms

1. The pectoralis major adducts the arms and shoulders across the chest.

2. The upper arm posterior deltoid contracts. This causes the upper arm to press down on the lower. The deltoid is contracting while in a stretched position, which is eccentric contraction. This action deepens the stretch of the rotator cuff in this pose.

3. The posterior deltoid of the lower arm is stretching while the anterior portion activates to press the lower elbow up, thus squeezing the elbows together.

4. The serratus anterior draws the scapulae forward, stretching the middle trapezius and rhomboids.

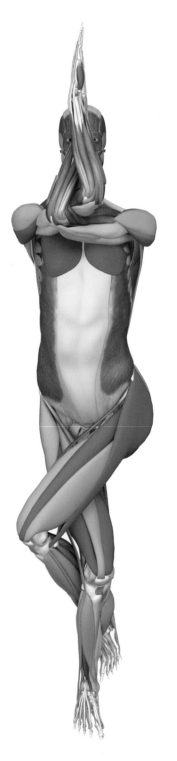

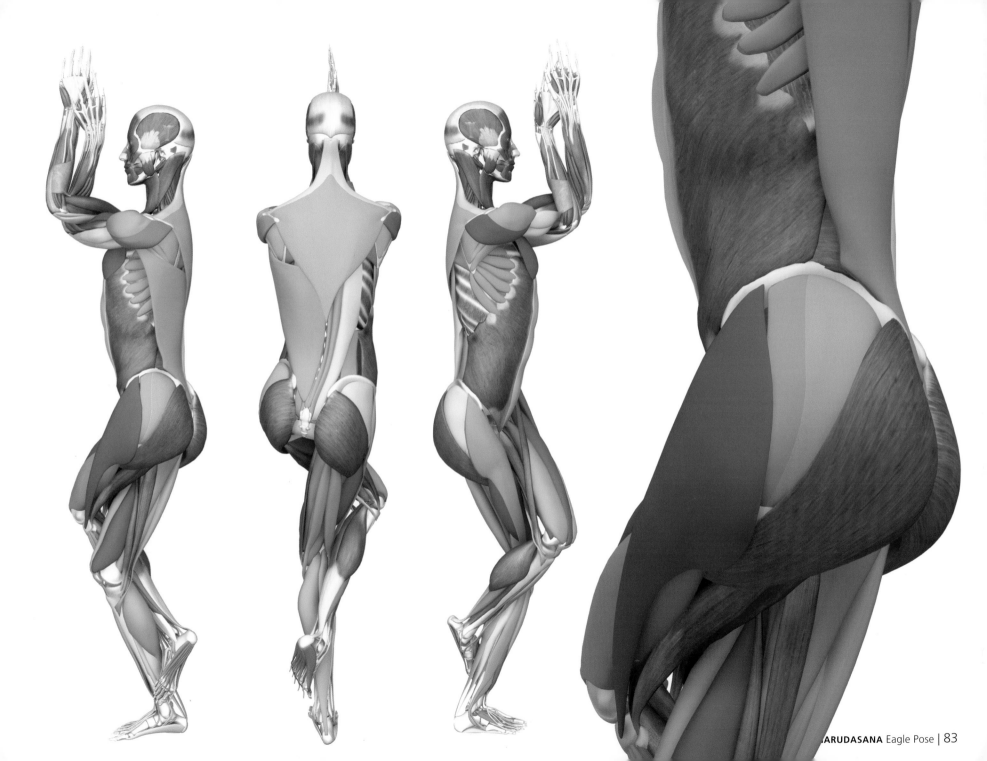

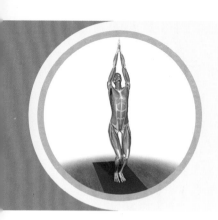

Utkatasana: Chair Pose

Utkatasana is a symmetrical standing pose and a natural progression from Mountain Pose, Tadasana. The stance, coiled as though preparing to jump, suggests potential energy to be unleashed. Utkatasana strengthens a number of the core muscle groups, including the muscles that flex the pelvis, the quadriceps, and the lower back muscles.

Synergizing/Activating

Pelvis and Legs

1. The hip flexors, including the psoas, pectineus, rectus femoris, and sartorius hold the femurs in a slightly flexed position. The gluteus maximus counters this action. This combination of flexion and extension of the pelvis stabilizes the pose.

2. The quadriceps are active, holding the knees in partial flexion.

3. The adductor group draws the knees together.

4. The tibialis anterior muscles draw the top of the feet toward the shin.

5. The gastrocnemius and soleus muscles eccentrically contract to ground the soles of the feet on the floor.

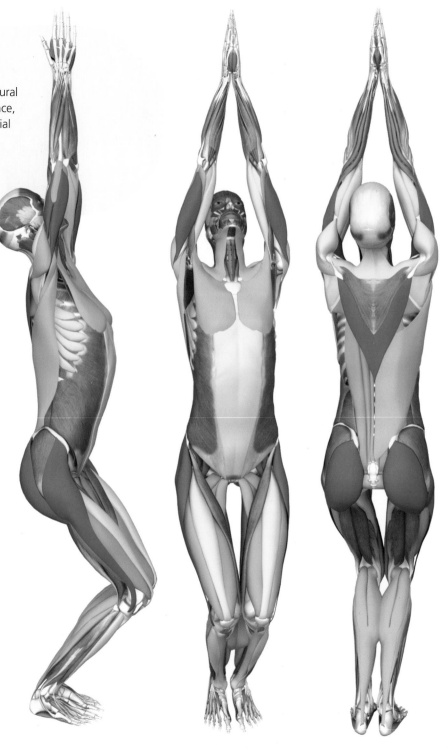

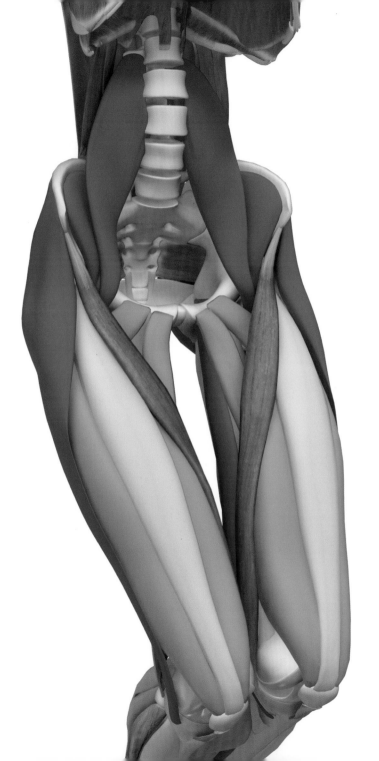

Trunk

1. The quadratus lumborum activates to arch the lower back. The erector spinae muscles synergize this action.

2. The psoas provides a counterbalance to the lower back muscles, aiding to protect the lumbar spine.

3. The rectus abdominis is active, tethering the rib cage to the pelvis and preventing the ribs from bulging forward in the pose.

Shoulders and Arms

1. The middle trapezius and rhomboids combine to draw the scapulae toward the midline of the back and open the chest.

2. The lower portion of the trapezius draws the shoulders away from the neck, freeing the cervical spine to extend.

3. The infraspinatus turns the shoulders outward.

4. The anterior deltoids activate to lift the arms over the head.

5. The triceps extend the elbows.

Hip Openers

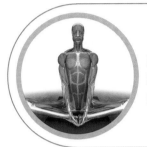

Baddha Konasana

Bound Angle Pose

Page 88

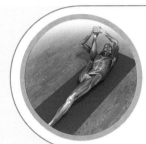

Supta Padangusthasana

Bent Knee Version

Page 90

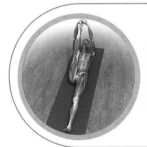

Supta Padangusthasana A

Sleeping Big Toe Pose

Page 92

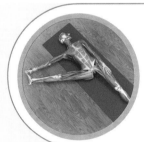

Supta Padangusthasana B

Sleeping Big Toe Pose

Page 94

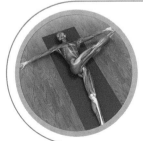

Supta Padangusthasana

(Revolving Variation)

Page 96

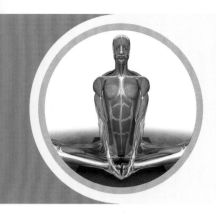

Baddha Konasana: Bound Angle Pose

Baddha Konasana connects the upper and lower appendicular skeletons by grasping (binding) the feet with the hands. The hips flex and turn outward, and the knees bend and move away from each other. This action stretches the adductor group of muscles along the inside of the thighs. The upper arms, shoulders, and back form a chain that links the hands and feet. Work with these structures to tighten the "bind" and deepen the pose.

Synergizing/Activating

1. The biceps brachii and brachialis (muscles down the front and inside of the upper arm) bend the elbows, drawing the feet upward and opening the pelvic region.

2. The lower and middle trapezius, which spans the back, and the rhomboids, muscles joining the shoulder blade to the spine, work together to draw the shoulders back and down, opening the chest.

3. The erector spinae muscles run the length of the spine, and the quadratus lumborum connects the back pelvis rib cage and spine. Together they lift the back. This force is transmitted to the shoulders and arms and is then connected to the feet.

4. The sartorius, tensor fascia lata, gluteus medius, and gluteus maximus turn the hips outward and lengthen the adductor muscles along the inner thigh.

5. The hamstrings bend the knees, lengthening the quadriceps along the front of the thigh. The deep external rotators of the hips turn the thighs outward.

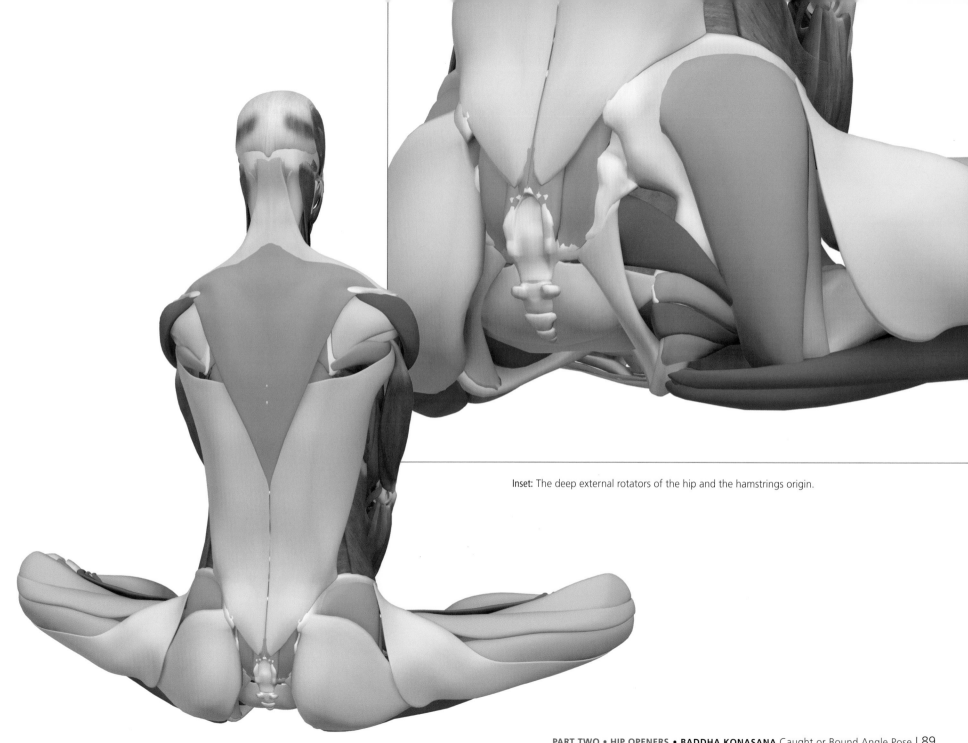

Inset: The deep external rotators of the hip and the hamstrings origin.

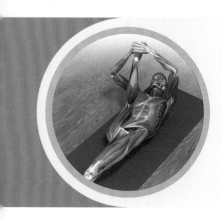

Supta Padangusthasana: Bent Knee Version

This version of the Sleeping Big Toe Pose has the knee of the stretching leg bent. This action focuses the stretch on the region where the gluteus maximus and the hamstrings, along the back of the thigh, are attached to the bones. Most of the stretch is accomplished by connecting the hands to the foot and using the force of the upper arms, shoulders, and back to draw the foot downwards.

Synergizing/Activating

Stretching Leg

1. The psoas, high at the top of the thigh, and the pectineus, attached to the thigh bone and the pubic bone, are activated, but they cannot generate much force when the hip is fully bent. Rather, they are used to align the hip joint and aid in the initial phase of the stretch.

2. The foot is drawn toward the chest by the biceps, the pectoralis major in the chest muscle, and the posterior deltoid, at the back of the shoulder.

3. The erector spinae, which flow the length of the spine, arch the back, intensifying the stretch.

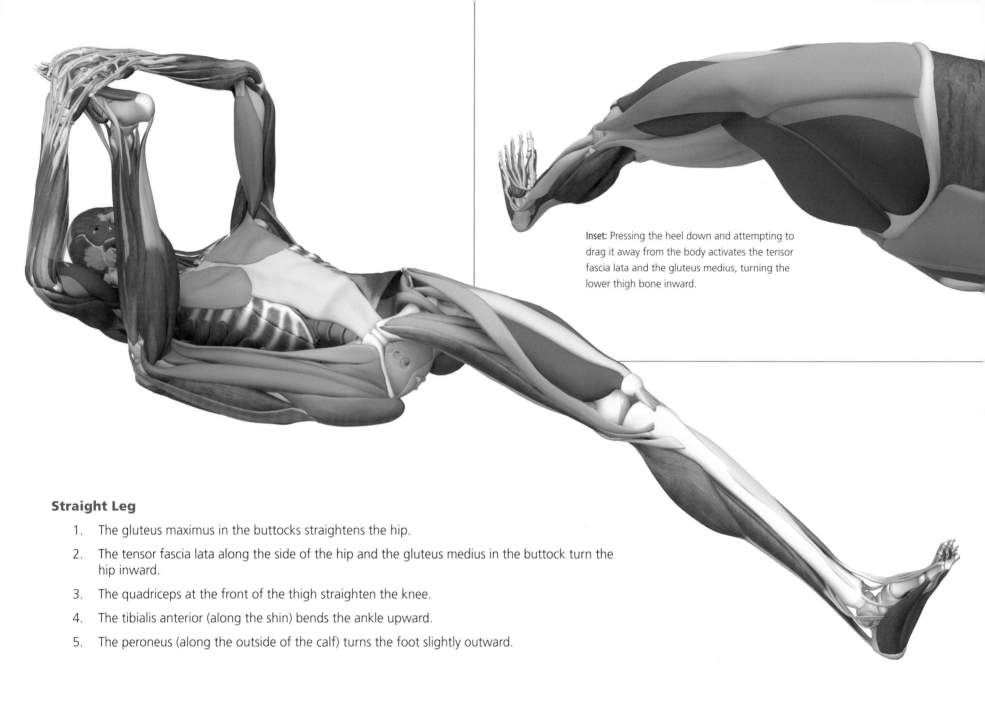

Inset: Pressing the heel down and attempting to drag it away from the body activates the tensor fascia lata and the gluteus medius, turning the lower thigh bone inward.

Straight Leg

1. The gluteus maximus in the buttocks straightens the hip.

2. The tensor fascia lata along the side of the hip and the gluteus medius in the buttock turn the hip inward.

3. The quadriceps at the front of the thigh straighten the knee.

4. The tibialis anterior (along the shin) bends the ankle upward.

5. The peroneus (along the outside of the calf) turns the foot slightly outward.

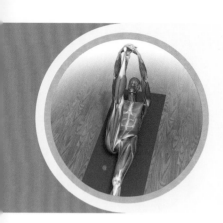

Supta Padangusthasana A: Sleeping Big Toe Pose

This is a variation on the reclining hip openers and is related to the standing pose Parsvottanasana. It is an intense stretch of the hamstrings down the back of the thigh and the gluteus maximus in the buttocks. It also involves an unusual form of activating the extensors and internal rotators that straighten and turn in the leg that remains on the floor.

Synergizing/Activating

Stretching Leg

1. The psoas at the top of the front of the thigh and the pectineus, attached to the thigh bone and pubic bone, flex the hip, stretching the gluteus maximus and the hamstrings along the back of that thigh.

2. The quadriceps straighten the knee, stretching the hamstrings behind.

Straight Leg

1. The hip is straightened by the gluteus maximus and also the gluteus medius, which is tucked partially under the buttocks.

2. The tensor fascia lata along the outside of the hip and gluteus medius in the buttocks turn the hip inward.

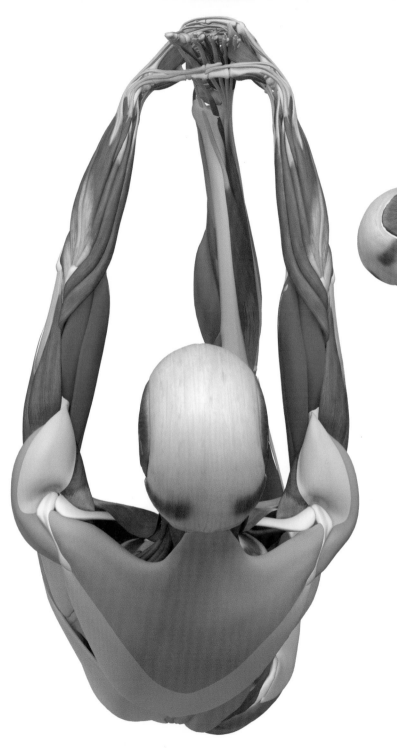

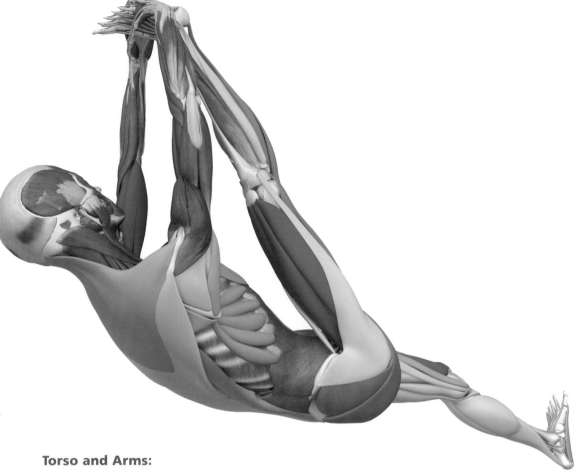

Torso and Arms:

1. The rectus abdominis, which flows from the chest to the pubic bone, bends the trunk.

2. The pectoralis major in the chest draws the arms toward the center line, pulling the leg to the chest.

3. The infraspinatus and teres minor over the shoulder blades turn the shoulders outward.

4. The lower trapezius (that spans the back) draws the shoulders away from the ears.

5. The biceps bend the elbows, drawing the leg toward the chest.

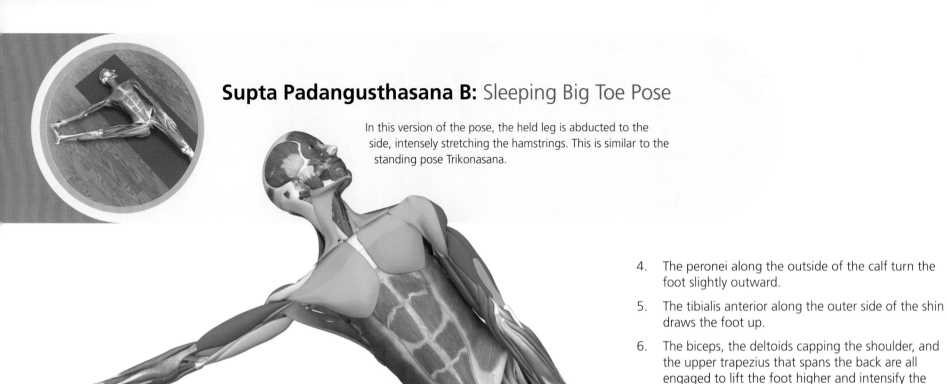

Supta Padangusthasana B: Sleeping Big Toe Pose

In this version of the pose, the held leg is abducted to the side, intensely stretching the hamstrings. This is similar to the standing pose Trikonasana.

4. The peronei along the outside of the calf turn the foot slightly outward.

5. The tibialis anterior along the outer side of the shin draws the foot up.

6. The biceps, the deltoids capping the shoulder, and the upper trapezius that spans the back are all engaged to lift the foot higher and intensify the stretch.

Synergizing/Activating

Stretching Leg

1. The psoas and pectineus bend the hip.

2. The sartorius, which runs diagonally across thigh, bends the hip, moves it away from the midline, and turns it outward.

3. The quadriceps straighten the knee.

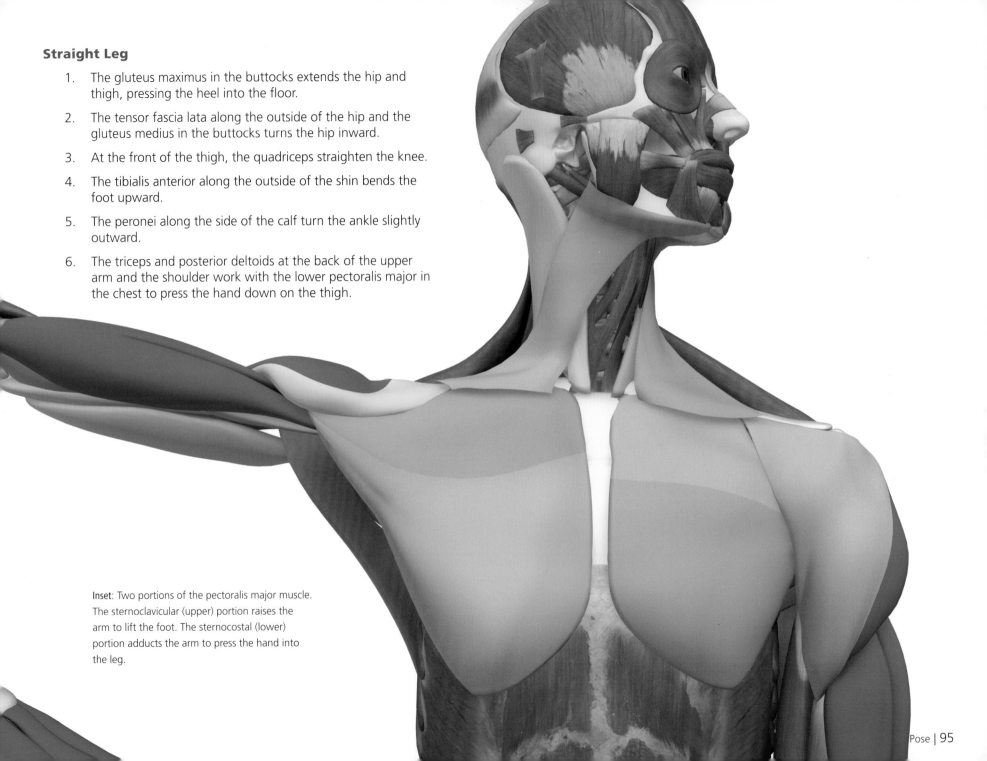

Straight Leg

1. The gluteus maximus in the buttocks extends the hip and thigh, pressing the heel into the floor.

2. The tensor fascia lata along the outside of the hip and the gluteus medius in the buttocks turns the hip inward.

3. At the front of the thigh, the quadriceps straighten the knee.

4. The tibialis anterior along the outside of the shin bends the foot upward.

5. The peronei along the side of the calf turn the ankle slightly outward.

6. The triceps and posterior deltoids at the back of the upper arm and the shoulder work with the lower pectoralis major in the chest to press the hand down on the thigh.

Inset: Two portions of the pectoralis major muscle. The sternoclavicular (upper) portion raises the arm to lift the foot. The sternocostal (lower) portion adducts the arm to press the hand into the leg.

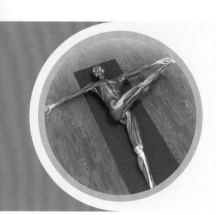

Supta Padangusthasana: Lying Down Big Toe Pose (Revolving Variation)

This is a variation of the Supta Padangusthasana pose and is related to Parivrtta Trikonasana. It affects many of the same muscle groups and is a combination of twist and hip opener.

Synergizing/Activating

1. The psoas (high at the front of the thigh) works with the pectineus, which is attached to the thigh bone and the pubic bone, and the rectus femoris down the front of the thigh to bend the upper hip.

2. The upper thigh bone is drawn toward the midline by the adductor longus and brevis of the inside thigh.

3. The tensor fascia lata on the outside of the hips and the anterior fibers of the gluteus medius in the buttocks work together to turn the thigh bone inward.

4. The quadriceps straighten the knees.

5. The lower hip is straightened by the gluteus maximus in the buttocks.

6. The adductor magnus on the inner thigh straightens the lower hip and draws the thigh bone toward the body.

7. The gluteus medius in the buttocks and tensor fascia lata along the outside of the hip work together to turn the thigh bone of the lower leg inward, thus counteracting the outward turning effects of the gluteus maximus.

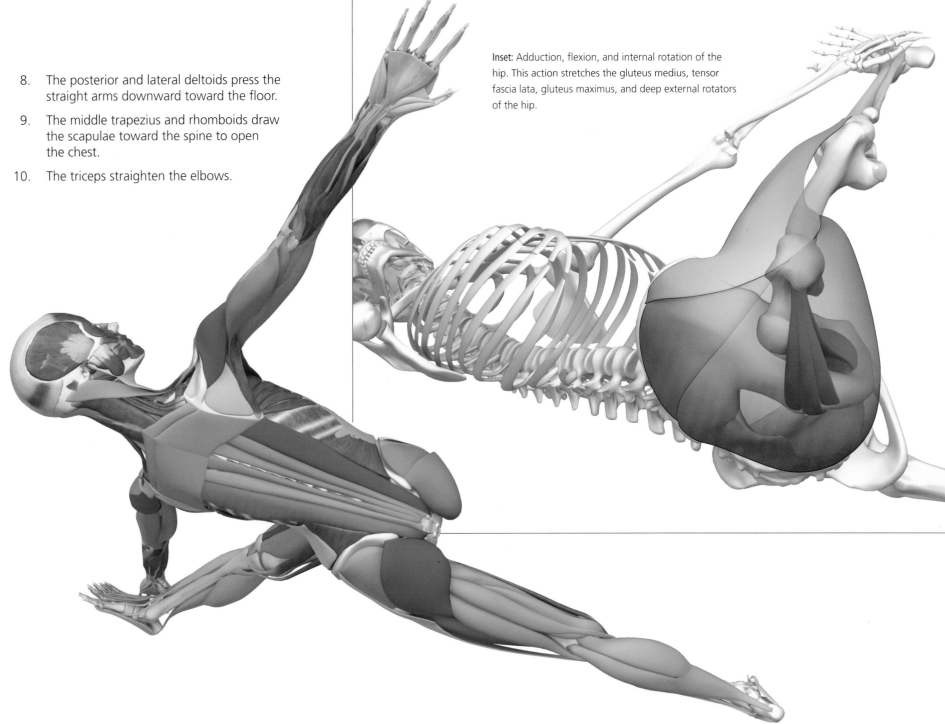

8. The posterior and lateral deltoids press the straight arms downward toward the floor.

9. The middle trapezius and rhomboids draw the scapulae toward the spine to open the chest.

10. The triceps straighten the elbows.

Inset: Adduction, flexion, and internal rotation of the hip. This action stretches the gluteus medius, tensor fascia lata, gluteus maximus, and deep external rotators of the hip.

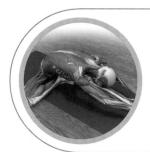
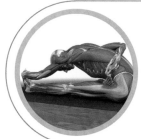
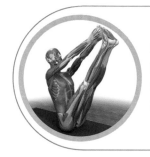

Forward Bends

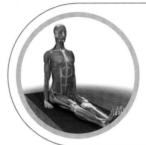

Dandasana
Staff Pose
Page 102

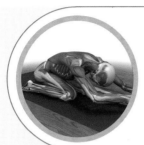

Trianga Mukhaikapada Paschimottanasana
Three Limbs Face One Foot Pose
Page 104

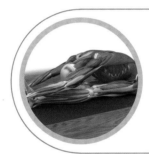

Paschimottanasana
Intense Stretch to the West
Page 108

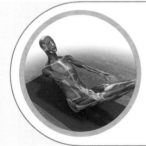

Navasana
Boat Pose
Page 110

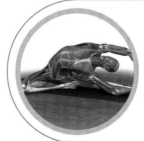

Parivrtta Janu Sirsasana
Revolving Head to Knee Pose
Page 114

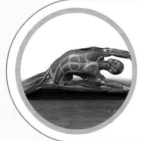

Parighasana
Cross Bar of the Gate Pose
Page 116

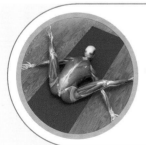

Kurmasana
Turtle Pose
Page 118

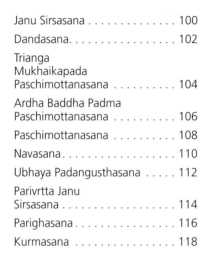

Janu Sirsasana: Head-to-Knee Pose

Janu Sirsasana is an asymmetric forward bend. It is similar to the hurdlers' stretch that athletes perform during warmup. This pose creates an intense stretch of the hamstrings in the straight leg. As with other poses that connect the upper and lower extremities, Janu Sirsasana also affects the lower back and shoulders. Focusing one's attention on the bent leg can be used to refine this pose.

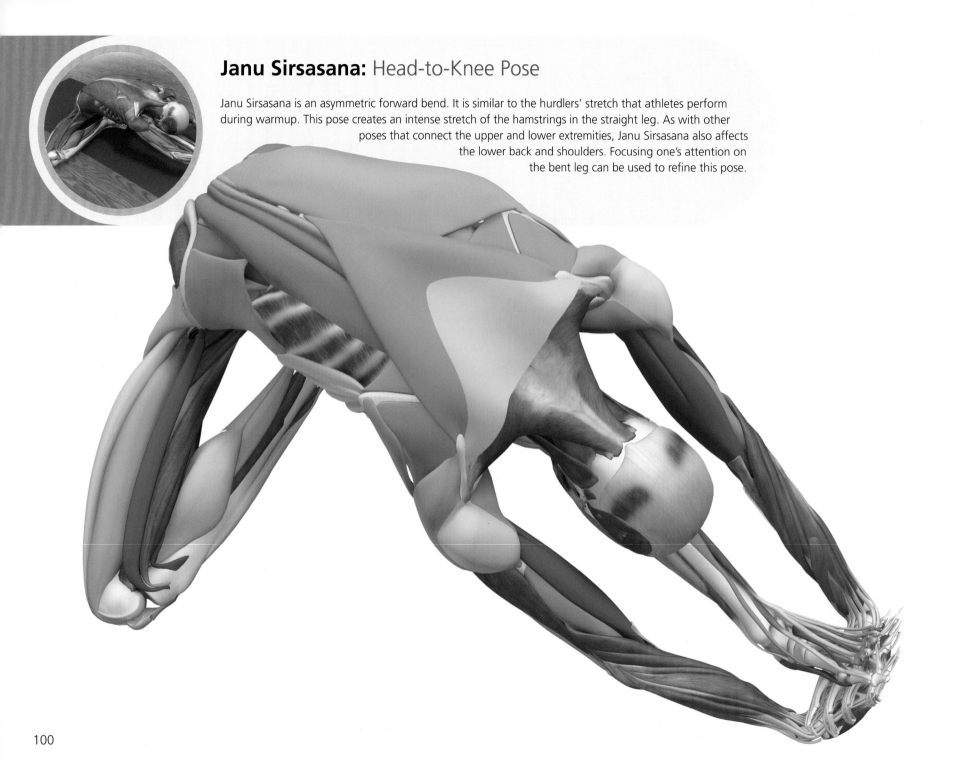

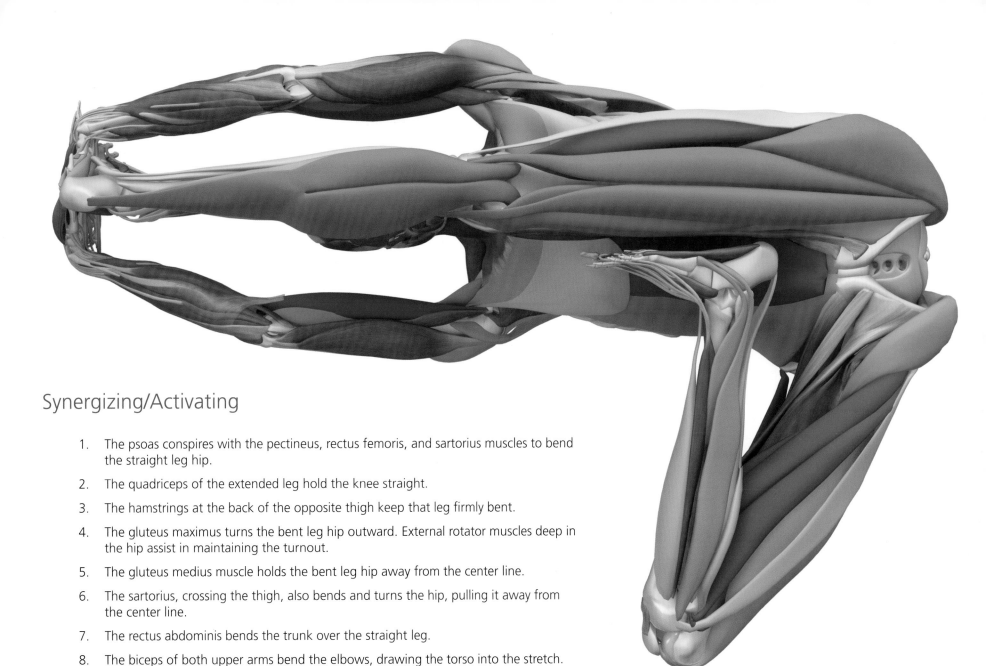

Synergizing/Activating

1. The psoas conspires with the pectineus, rectus femoris, and sartorius muscles to bend the straight leg hip.

2. The quadriceps of the extended leg hold the knee straight.

3. The hamstrings at the back of the opposite thigh keep that leg firmly bent.

4. The gluteus maximus turns the bent leg hip outward. External rotator muscles deep in the hip assist in maintaining the turnout.

5. The gluteus medius muscle holds the bent leg hip away from the center line.

6. The sartorius, crossing the thigh, also bends and turns the hip, pulling it away from the center line.

7. The rectus abdominis bends the trunk over the straight leg.

8. The biceps of both upper arms bend the elbows, drawing the torso into the stretch.

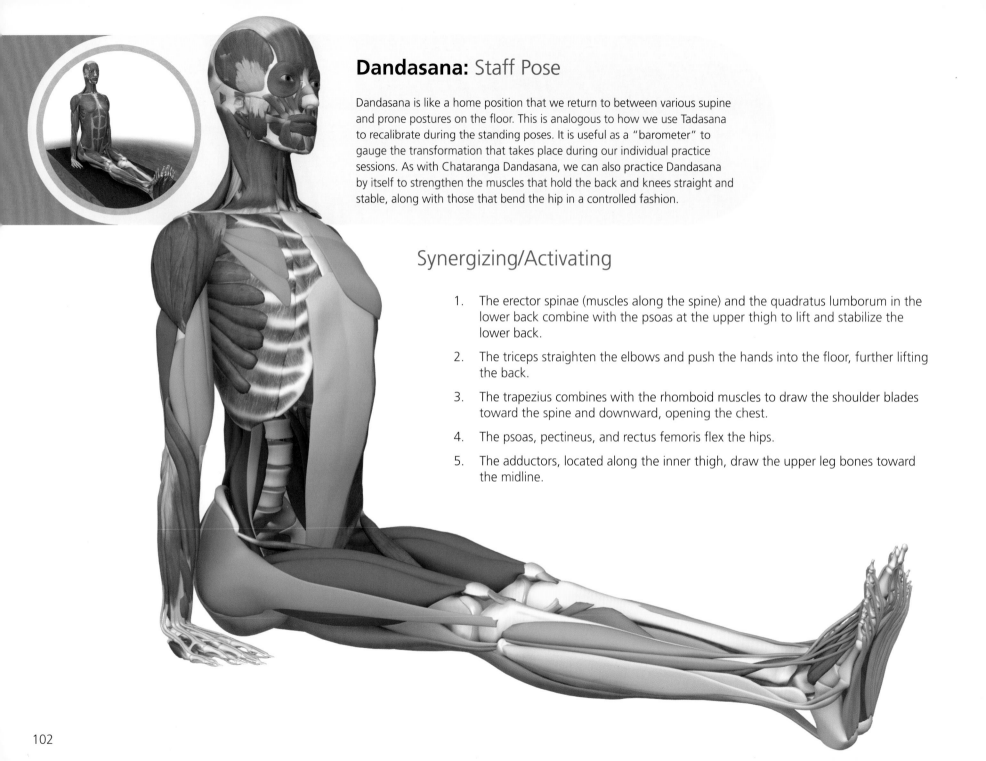

Dandasana: Staff Pose

Dandasana is like a home position that we return to between various supine and prone postures on the floor. This is analogous to how we use Tadasana to recalibrate during the standing poses. It is useful as a "barometer" to gauge the transformation that takes place during our individual practice sessions. As with Chataranga Dandasana, we can also practice Dandasana by itself to strengthen the muscles that hold the back and knees straight and stable, along with those that bend the hip in a controlled fashion.

Synergizing/Activating

1. The erector spinae (muscles along the spine) and the quadratus lumborum in the lower back combine with the psoas at the upper thigh to lift and stabilize the lower back.

2. The triceps straighten the elbows and push the hands into the floor, further lifting the back.

3. The trapezius combines with the rhomboid muscles to draw the shoulder blades toward the spine and downward, opening the chest.

4. The psoas, pectineus, and rectus femoris flex the hips.

5. The adductors, located along the inner thigh, draw the upper leg bones toward the midline.

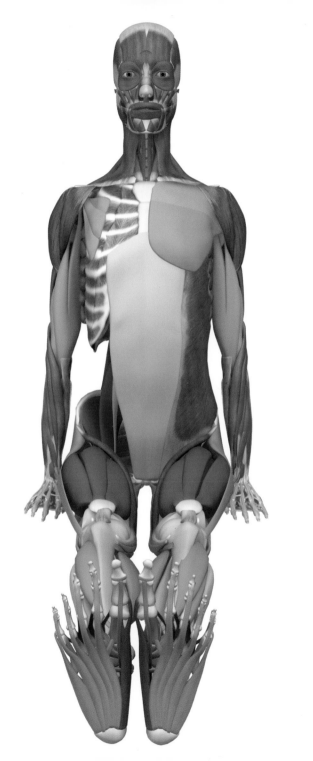

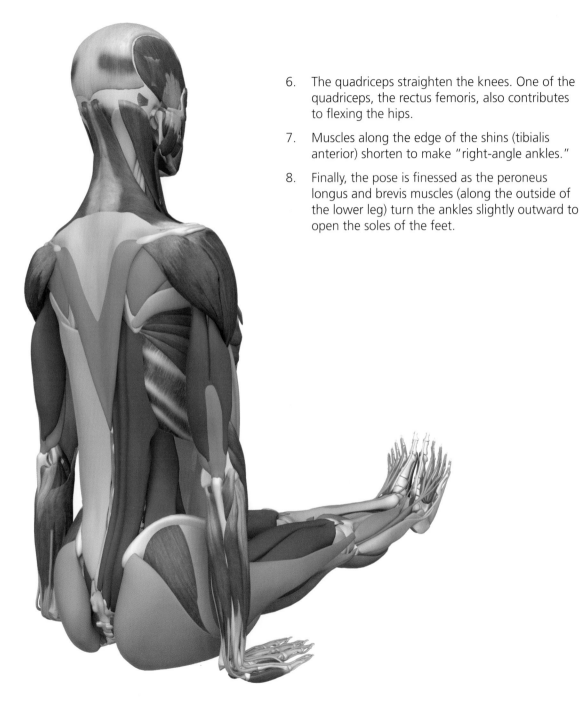

6. The quadriceps straighten the knees. One of the quadriceps, the rectus femoris, also contributes to flexing the hips.

7. Muscles along the edge of the shins (tibialis anterior) shorten to make "right-angle ankles."

8. Finally, the pose is finessed as the peroneus longus and brevis muscles (along the outside of the lower leg) turn the ankles slightly outward to open the soles of the feet.

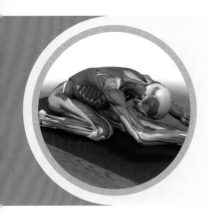

Trianga Mukhaikapada Paschimottanasana:
Three Limbs Face One Foot Pose

This pose is an asymmetrical forward bend; that is, one leg is bent. Like the poses that use both sides of the body at the same time, asymmetrical poses show us where we need to improve in order to move toward symmetry. The tendency in this pose is to fall over toward the straight-leg side. Activating the psoas and the hamstrings of the bent leg draws the body back over the bent leg. In this way, we can use the asymmetry of the pose to awaken these muscles.

Synergizing/Activating

Bent Leg

1. The hamstrings at the back of the thigh bend the knee, drawing the body toward the bent leg. The gastrocnemius in the calf assists the hamstrings in bending the knee.

2. The psoas bends the hip and opposes the tendency to fall over the straight leg by drawing the body toward the bent-leg side.

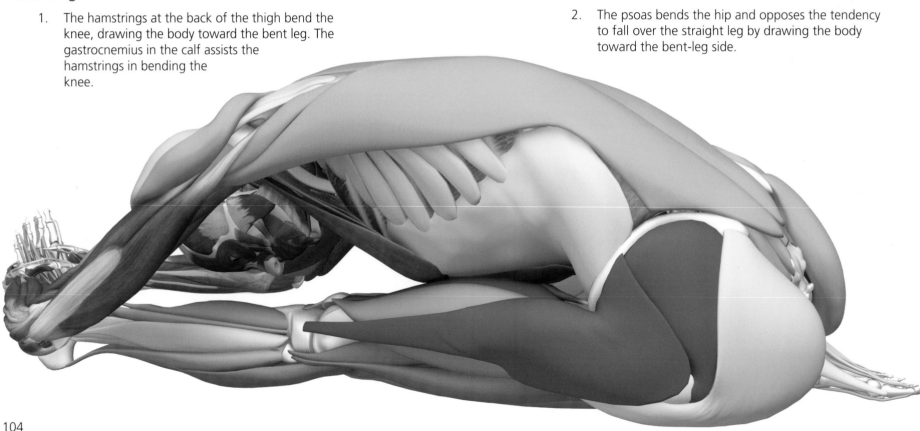

Stretching Leg

1. The psoas bends the hip.

2. The gluteus medius and the tensor fascia lata activate to turn the hip inward, rolling the body toward the bent knee.

3. The quadriceps straighten the knee.

4. The adductor group, on the inside of the thigh, draws the thigh toward the bent-leg side.

Trunk

1. The abdominals activate to bend the trunk.

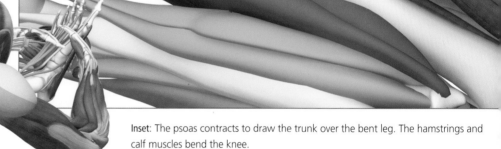

Inset: The psoas contracts to draw the trunk over the bent leg. The hamstrings and calf muscles bend the knee.

2. Actively flexing the trunk creates reciprocal inhibition of the back extensors, allowing them to lengthen.

Shoulders and Arms

1. The biceps bend the elbows, drawing the torso toward the straight leg.

2. The deltoids lift the shoulders.

3. The middle trapezius, which spans the back, combines with the rhomboids to draw the scapulae toward the spine.

4. The lower trapezius draws the shoulders away from the neck.

Ardha Baddha Padma Paschimottanasana:
Half-Bound Lotus Forward Bend

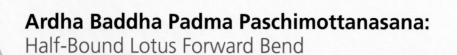

This pose binds the shoulder to the opposite hip. Bending the torso forward over the straight leg stretches the muscles at the back of the thigh, hip, and back. As a half-lotus, it is considered asymmetrical and is useful for identifying differences between the two sides of the body.

Synergizing/Activating

1. The pectoralis, a fan-shaped muscle attached to the breastbone and collarbone, and the subscapularis, a triangular muscle stretching from the shoulder blade, converge on the bone in the upper arm to turn the shoulder on the bent-leg side up behind the back and inward. This stretches two other muscles, the infraspinatus and teres minor, each connected to the shoulder blade and the upper arm bone.

2. The posterior deltoid, teres major, and latissimus dorsi are muscles located at the back of the shoulder and down the rib cage. These muscles attach to the bone in the upper arm. They work together to extend the shoulder and arm, allowing the hand to grasp the foot of the half-lotus leg. At the same time, the muscles at the back of the extended arm, the deltoids, are engaged to create a pull on the grasped foot, thus deepening the pose and stretching the quadriceps.

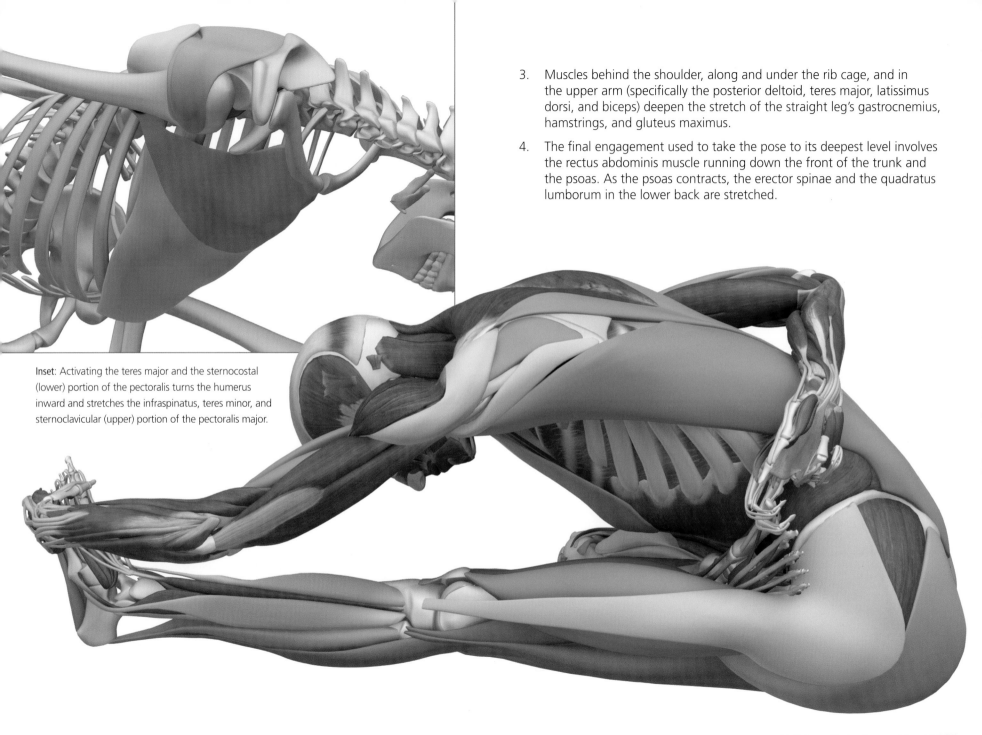

3. Muscles behind the shoulder, along and under the rib cage, and in the upper arm (specifically the posterior deltoid, teres major, latissimus dorsi, and biceps) deepen the stretch of the straight leg's gastrocnemius, hamstrings, and gluteus maximus.

4. The final engagement used to take the pose to its deepest level involves the rectus abdominis muscle running down the front of the trunk and the psoas. As the psoas contracts, the erector spinae and the quadratus lumborum in the lower back are stretched.

Inset: Activating the teres major and the sternocostal (lower) portion of the pectoralis turns the humerus inward and stretches the infraspinatus, teres minor, and sternoclavicular (upper) portion of the pectoralis major.

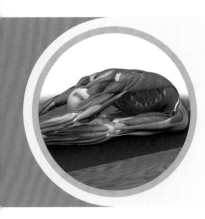

Paschimottanasana: Intense Stretch to the West

This pose is a symmetrical forward bend that intensely and evenly stretches the calf muscles, the muscles down the back of the thigh, the large buttock muscles, and the muscles that run down the length of the spine. The upper extremities connect to the lower extremities to transmit the force of the stretch to the spine and trunk. In other words, the hands grasp the feet of the outstretched legs and gently pull, helping to fold the torso.

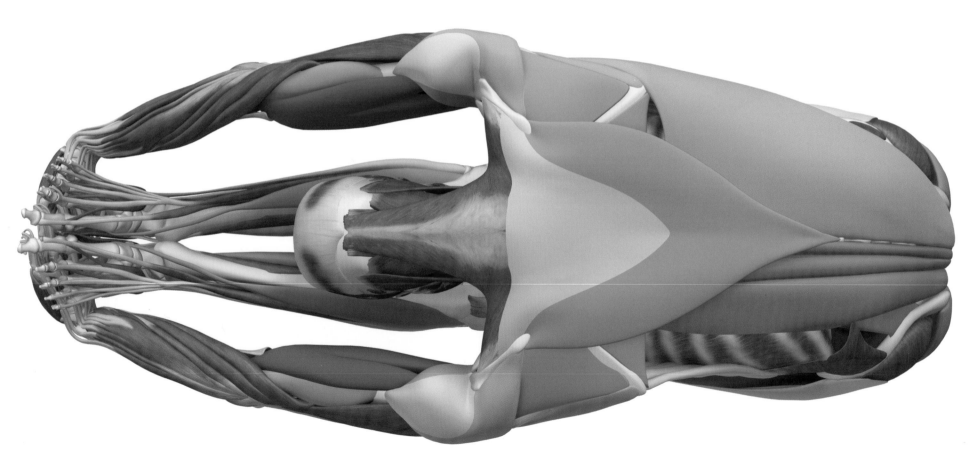

Synergizing/Activating

1. The hips are bent by the psoas, pectineus, rectus femoris, and sartorius muscles connecting the thigh bones and pelvis.

2. The adductor group draws the thighs together.

3. The quadriceps straighten the knees, stretching the hamstrings. The act of contracting the quadriceps initiates reciprocal inhibition, causing the hamstrings to relax.

4. The ankles are bent upward by the tibialis anterior muscles along the front of the shins, stretching the muscles on the back of the calf.

5. The peroneus muscles along the outside of the calf turn the ankle slightly outward, opening the soles of the feet.

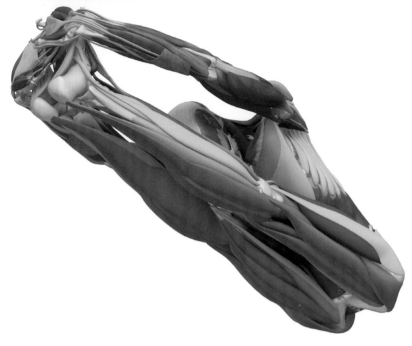

Inset: Intense stretch of the calf muscles, hamstrings, and gluteus maximus.

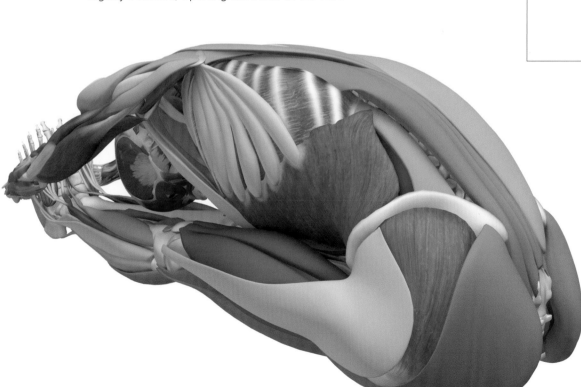

6. The rectus abdominis muscle flows from the chest to the pubic bone and bends the trunk toward the knees, stretching the back muscles.

7. The biceps bend the elbows slightly to draw the torso farther over the thighs, intensifying the stretch.

8. The infraspinatus and teres minor muscles located over the shoulder blades turn the shoulders gently outward to further flatten the upper body against the thighs.

9. The rhomboids and middle trapezius draw the shoulder blades toward the spine, opening the chest.

10. The lower trapezius muscles that span the back draw the shoulders away from the neck.

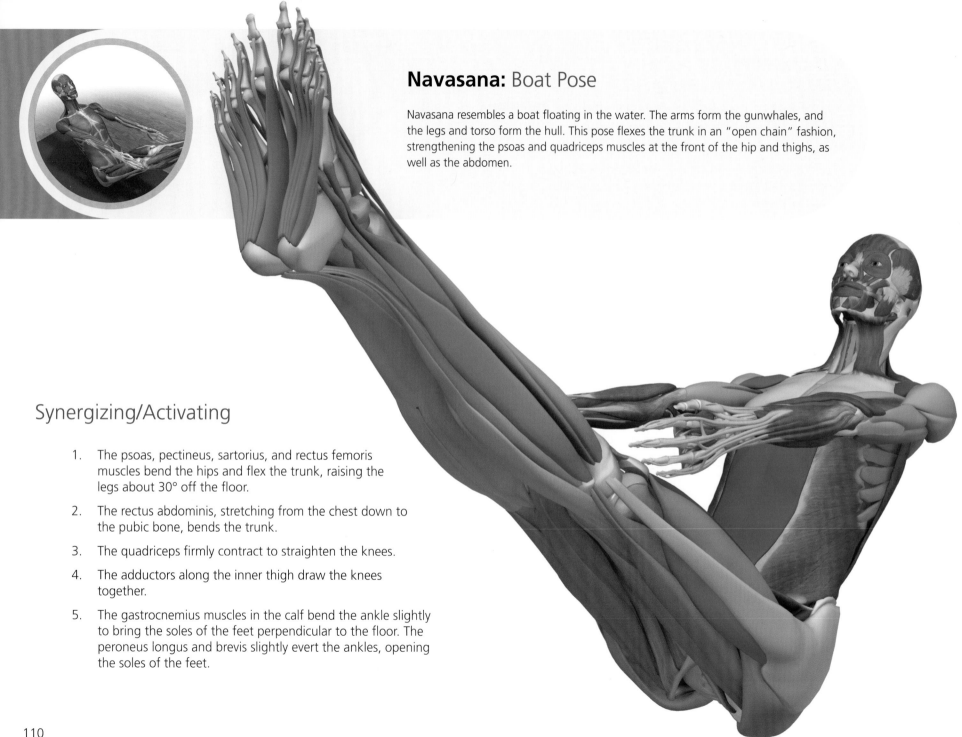

Navasana: Boat Pose

Navasana resembles a boat floating in the water. The arms form the gunwhales, and the legs and torso form the hull. This pose flexes the trunk in an "open chain" fashion, strengthening the psoas and quadriceps muscles at the front of the hip and thighs, as well as the abdomen.

Synergizing/Activating

1. The psoas, pectineus, sartorius, and rectus femoris muscles bend the hips and flex the trunk, raising the legs about 30° off the floor.

2. The rectus abdominis, stretching from the chest down to the pubic bone, bends the trunk.

3. The quadriceps firmly contract to straighten the knees.

4. The adductors along the inner thigh draw the knees together.

5. The gastrocnemius muscles in the calf bend the ankle slightly to bring the soles of the feet perpendicular to the floor. The peroneus longus and brevis slightly evert the ankles, opening the soles of the feet.

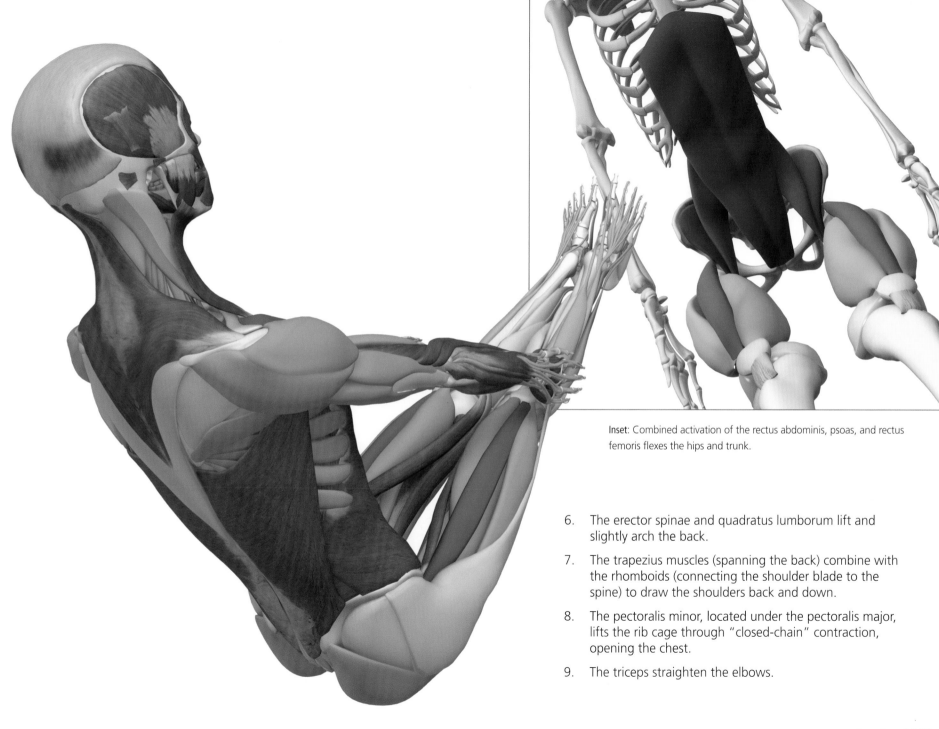

Inset: Combined activation of the rectus abdominis, psoas, and rectus femoris flexes the hips and trunk.

6. The erector spinae and quadratus lumborum lift and slightly arch the back.

7. The trapezius muscles (spanning the back) combine with the rhomboids (connecting the shoulder blade to the spine) to draw the shoulders back and down.

8. The pectoralis minor, located under the pectoralis major, lifts the rib cage through "closed-chain" contraction, opening the chest.

9. The triceps straighten the elbows.

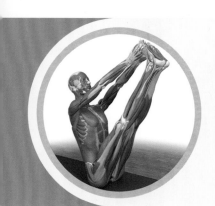

Ubhaya Padangusthasana: Both Feet Big Toe Pose

Ubhaya Padangusthasana, sometimes known as Jumping in With Both Feet, combines a forward bend and balancing pose. It connects the upper and lower extremities and uses the arms and shoulders to deepen the pose.

Synergizing/Activating

Shoulders and Arms

1. The biceps bend the elbows, drawing the legs toward the body.

2. The rhomboids, connected to the spine and the shoulder blades, work with the middle trapezius (spanning the back) to draw the shoulder blades (or scapulae) toward the midline, opening the chest.

3. The latissimus dorsi and teres major around the shoulders contract to lift the chest.

4. The lower trapezius muscles draw the shoulders down the back.

5. The infraspinatus and teres minor muscles turn the shoulder outward.

Trunk

1. The abdominals contract to bend the trunk.

2. The erector spinae and the quadratus lumborum in the lumbar spine activate, creating a slight arch in the back.

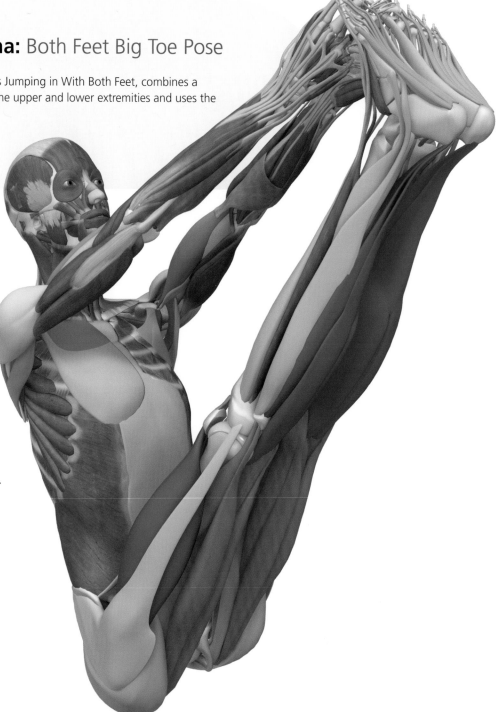

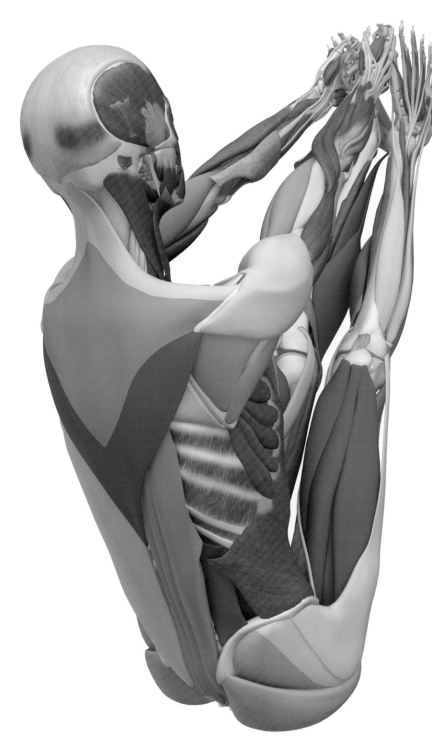

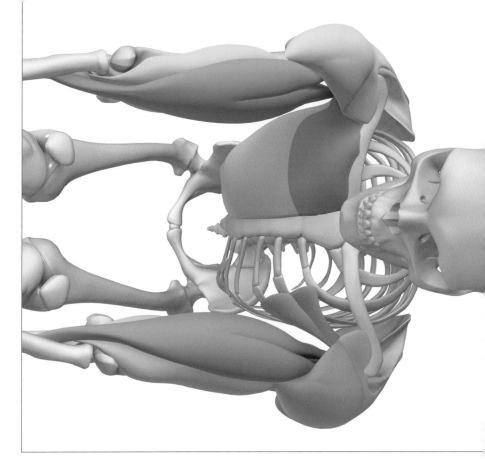

Inset: Activation of the pectorals (minor and major) lifts the chest. The biceps synergize with the hip flexors. This is an example of connecting the upper and lower appendicular skeletons to deepen a pose.

Pelvis and Legs

1. The psoas and the pectineus (attached to the thigh bone and pubic bone) bend the hips.

2. The quadriceps (along the front of the thighs) straighten the legs.

3. The gastrocnemius and soleus (calf muscles) bend the feet downward to "lock" the grip of the hands.

4. The peronei along the outside of the calf turn the feet out slightly.

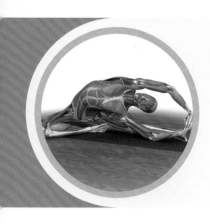

Parivrtta Janu Sirsasana:
Revolving Head to Knee Pose

This pose resembles Parighasana but differs in that the bended leg is placed in a manner similar to Janu Sirsasana. The knee can be abducted progressively, or drawn further backward, to intensify the stretch of the adductor group of muscles on the inside of the thigh.

Synergizing/Activating

1. The quadriceps extend the knee of the straight leg.

2. The psoas combines with the pectineus, rectus femoris, and sartorius to bend the hip of the straight leg.

3. The tensor fascia lata down the outside of the straight leg hip maintains the straight leg in a neutral position with the kneecap facing upward.

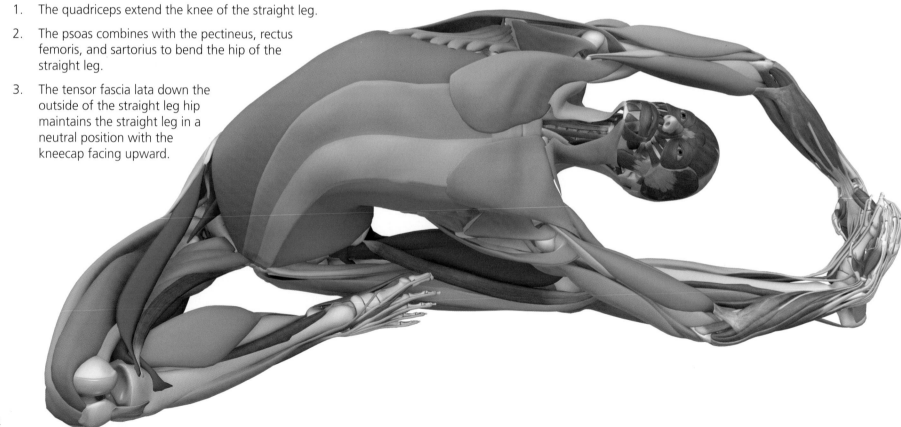

4. In the bent leg, the sartorius muscle pulls the calf closer to the thigh, moves the knee farther from the midline, and turns the leg outward.

5. The bent hip is also moved away from the midline by the gluteus medius and the tensor fascia lata, abducting it and stretching the muscles on the inside of the thigh.

6. The bent-leg gluteus maximus in the buttocks extends and turns the hip outward.

7. The peroneus longus and brevis down the outside of the calf turn the ankle of the straight leg slightly outward. These same muscles are gently stretched in the bent leg by inverting the foot to turn the sole slightly upward.

8. The anterior deltoids at the front of the shoulders lift the humeri away from the torso, opening the chest.

9. The biceps activate to bend the elbows, drawing the torso toward the straight leg.

10. The infraspinatus and teres minor muscles rotate the humerus to refine the pose.

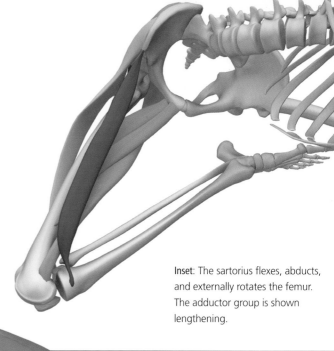

Inset: The sartorius flexes, abducts, and externally rotates the femur. The adductor group is shown lengthening.

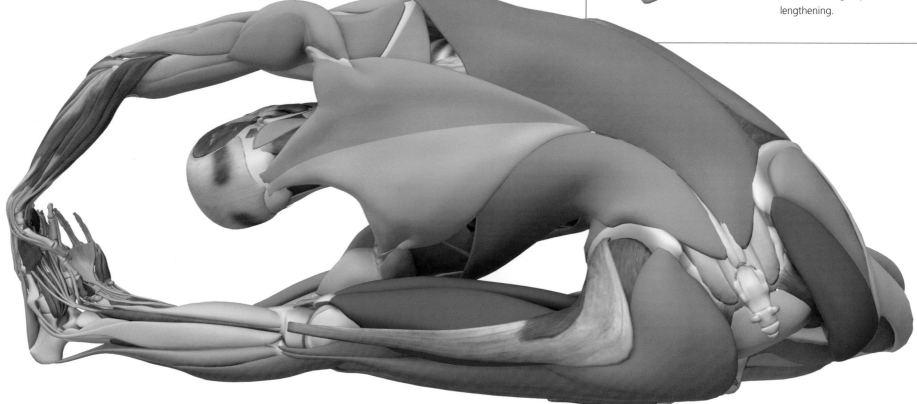

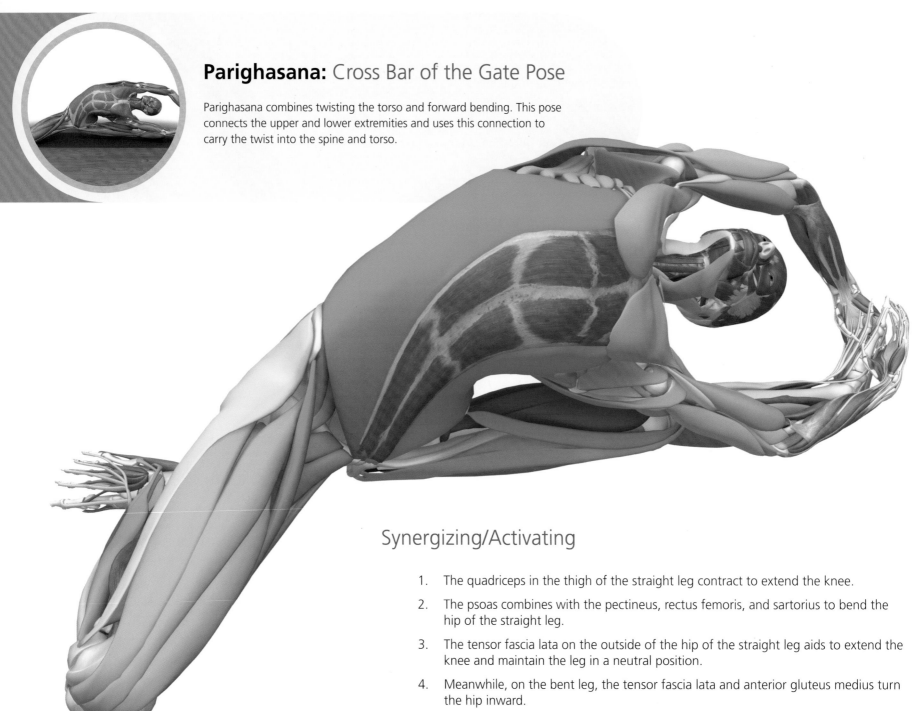

Parighasana: Cross Bar of the Gate Pose

Parighasana combines twisting the torso and forward bending. This pose connects the upper and lower extremities and uses this connection to carry the twist into the spine and torso.

Synergizing/Activating

1. The quadriceps in the thigh of the straight leg contract to extend the knee.

2. The psoas combines with the pectineus, rectus femoris, and sartorius to bend the hip of the straight leg.

3. The tensor fascia lata on the outside of the hip of the straight leg aids to extend the knee and maintain the leg in a neutral position.

4. Meanwhile, on the bent leg, the tensor fascia lata and anterior gluteus medius turn the hip inward.

5. The bent leg's gluteus maximus extends the hip away from the body.

6. The peroneus longus and brevis along the outside of the legs turn the ankles out slightly.

7. The anterior deltoids and the biceps activate to open the chest, with the lower elbow pressing into the knee to turn the torso.

8. The infraspinatus muscle turns the upper arm bone outward to refine the pose.

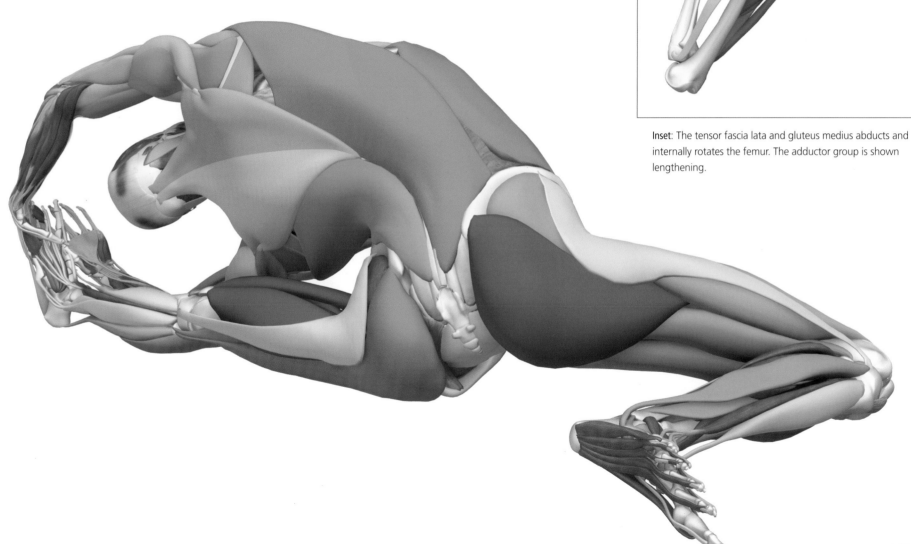

Inset: The tensor fascia lata and gluteus medius abducts and internally rotates the femur. The adductor group is shown lengthening.

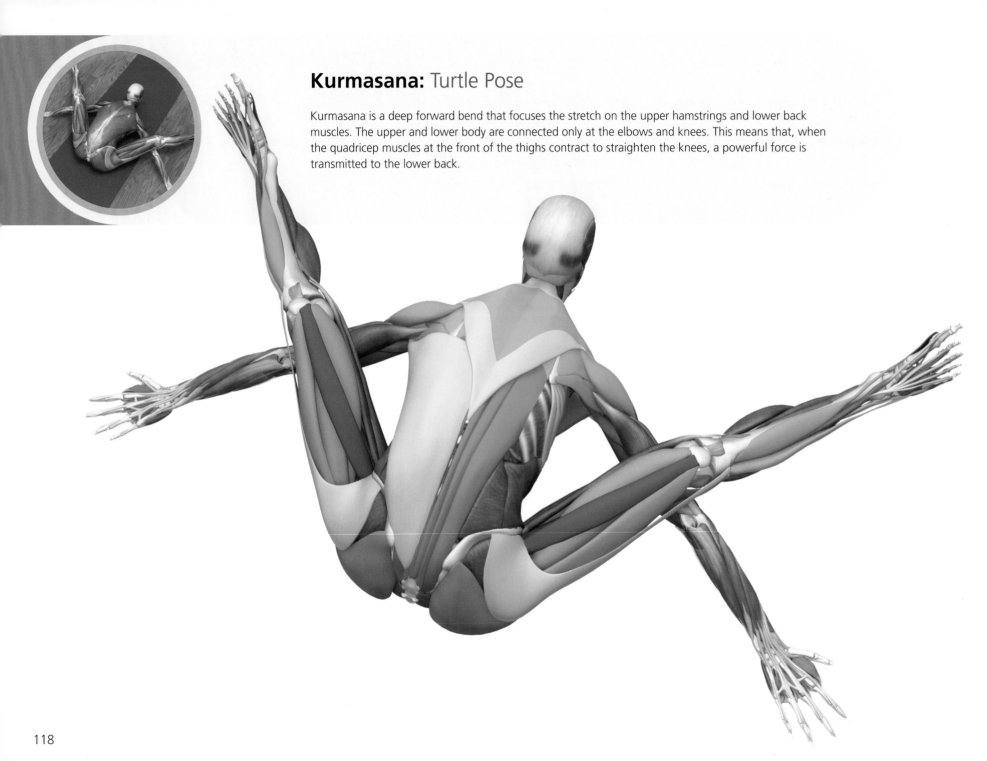

Kurmasana: Turtle Pose

Kurmasana is a deep forward bend that focuses the stretch on the upper hamstrings and lower back muscles. The upper and lower body are connected only at the elbows and knees. This means that, when the quadricep muscles at the front of the thighs contract to straighten the knees, a powerful force is transmitted to the lower back.

Synergizing/Activating

1. The quadriceps straighten the knees and press the elbows down. This creates a direct stretch of the hamstring muscles below the buttocks and an indirect stretch of the erector spinae and quadratus lumborum in the lower back.

2. The biceps and anterior deltoids at the front of the shoulder, as well as the pectoralis major in the chest, contract in the initial phase of the poses and then relax as the back muscles stretch and one goes deeper.

3. The posterior deltoids at the back of the shoulder stretch out the shoulders to deepen the pose as the triceps straighten the elbows.

4. The psoas muscles high at the front of the thigh bend the hips.

5. The tibialis anterior (along the outside shin) bends the ankles toward the shins and the peronei evert the ankles, opening the soles of the feet.

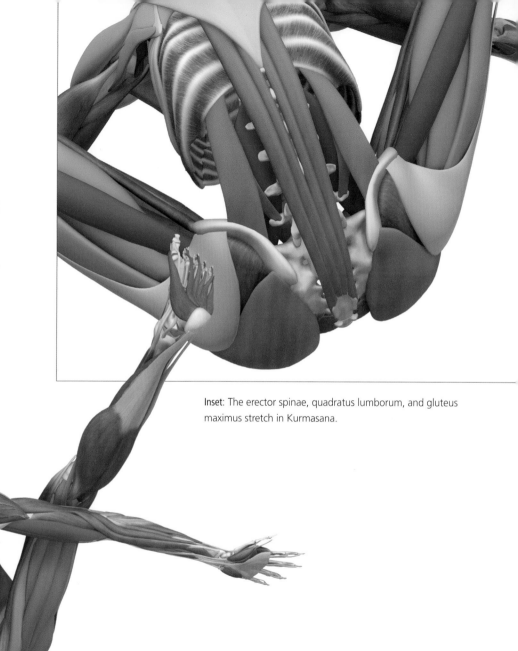

Inset: The erector spinae, quadratus lumborum, and gluteus maximus stretch in Kurmasana.

Twists

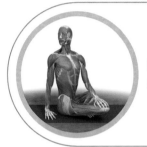

Seated Twist
Page 122

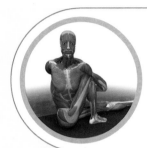

Marichyasana III
Great Sage Pose
Page 124

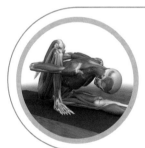

Marichyasana I
Great Sage Pose
Page 126

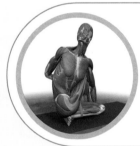

Ardha Matsyendrasana
Lord of the Fishes Pose
Page 128

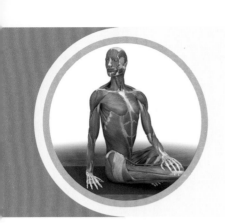

Seated Twist

This twist can be used as a preparation pose or to gently release tightness that may accumulate from back bends or forward bends.

Synergizing/Activating

1. The erector spinae and the quadratus lumborum lift the torso, slightly arching the back.

2. The latissimus dorsi, posterior deltoid, and triceps work in concert with the abdominals to turn the trunk.

3. To turn the body to the same side, the biceps, upper pectoralis in the chest, and anterior deltoids at the front of the shoulder work together to turn the trunk.

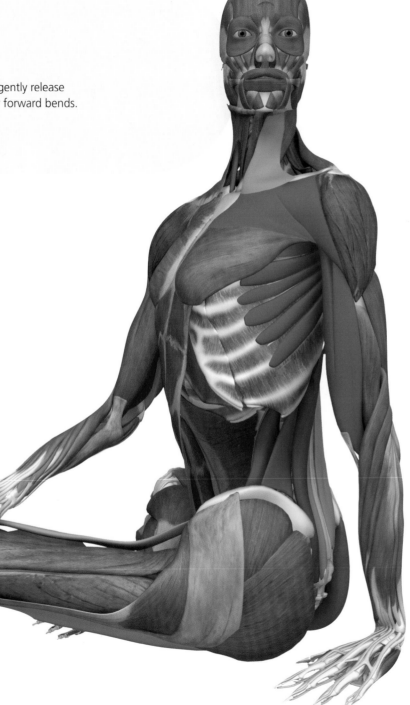

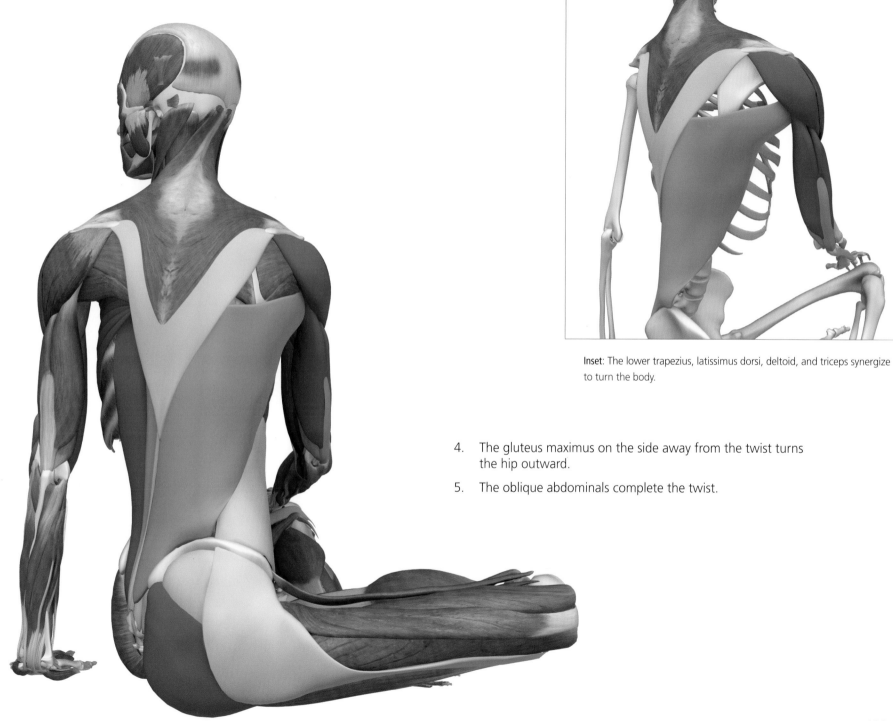

Inset: The lower trapezius, latissimus dorsi, deltoid, and triceps synergize to turn the body.

4. The gluteus maximus on the side away from the twist turns the hip outward.

5. The oblique abdominals complete the twist.

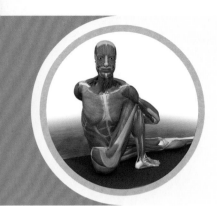

Marichyasana III: Great Sage Pose

Marichyasana III is a twist that involves the upper body turning out and the lower body turning in. This means that muscles with a rotatory component can be put to further use in order to deepen and refine the pose. For example, contracting the deep muscles that turn the thigh bone out on the bent-leg side can refine the twist. These include the external rotators of the hip and the gluteus maximus.

Synergizing/Activating

1. The posterior deltoids extend the shoulders back away from the body, stretching the anterior deltoids.

2. The triceps work to extend the elbows away from the body.

3. The lower trapezius, spanning the back, draws the shoulders away from the neck.

4. The middle trapezius works with the rhomboid muscles, joining the shoulder blade and the spine to draw the shoulders back toward the midline, opening the chest.

5. The pectoralis minor chest muscle lifts the lower rib cage.

6. The oblique abdominals activate to increase the twist of the torso.

7. The psoas and pectineus flex the bent leg at the hip.

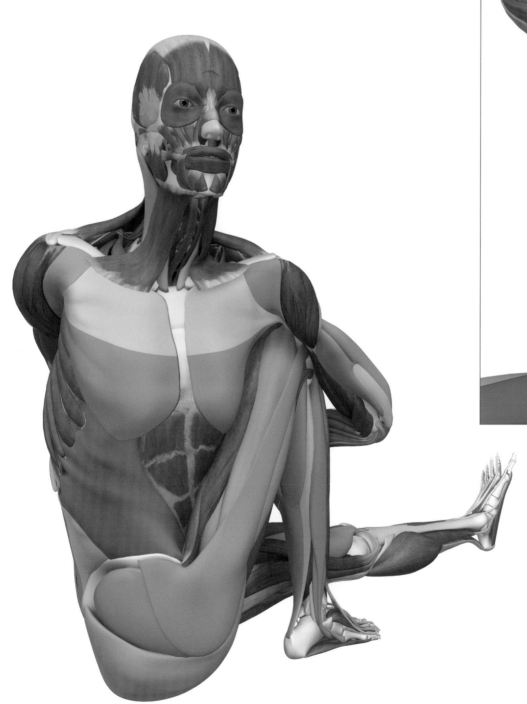

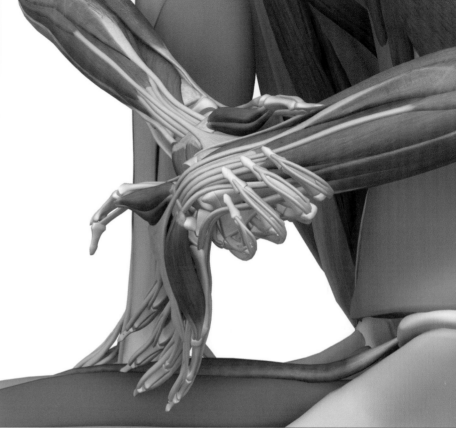

Inset: The wrist extensors bend the wrist to create a lock with the grasping hand.

8. The gluteus medius and tensor fascia lata (deep in the buttocks of the bent leg and along the side of the hip) turn the thigh bone inward. Both of these muscles move the hip away from the center line, abducting it. This action presses the outer part of the knee against the arm, deepening the turn.

9. The hamstrings on the outer side of the bent knee (biceps femoris) activate to rotate the hip.

10. The quadriceps of the extended leg straighten the knee, and the tibialis anterior muscle (along the outside of the shin) bends the foot toward the shin.

11. The peroneus longus and brevis evert the ankle and turn the foot slightly outward, opening the sole of the foot.

Marichyasana I: Great Sage Pose

Marichyasana I turns the body in the opposite direction of Marichyasana III. It involves the upper body turning inward, while the lower body turns outward. This means that muscles with a turning capacity can be activated to deepen and refine the pose. These include the rotator cuff, the rotators of the hip, and the inner and outer hamstrings.

Synergizing/Activating

1. The pectoralis major of the chest and subscapularis muscle under the shoulder blade turn the shoulders inward and stretch the infraspinatus and teres minor.

2. The triceps muscles work to straighten the elbows, thus deepening the torso flexing forward.

3. The deep external rotators of the bent-leg hip turn the thigh bone outward, while the gluteus medius and tensor fascia lata press the knee into the arm.

4. The inner hamstrings of the bent leg rotate the tibia inward. The net effect of this action turns the hip outward, in a direction opposite to the torso.

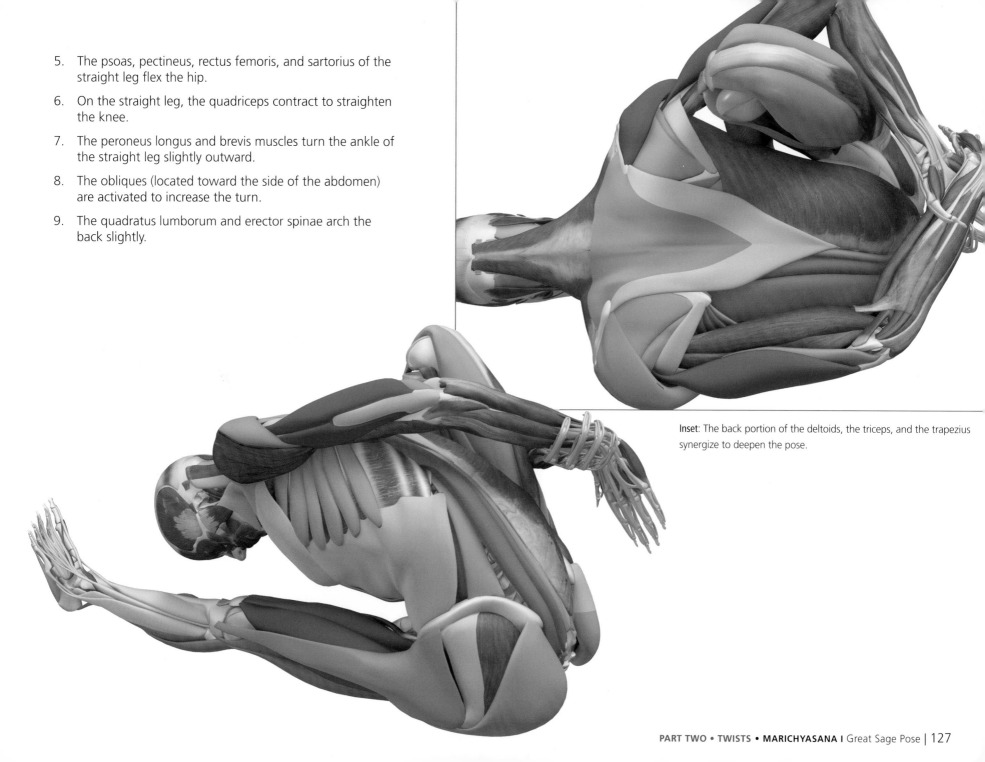

5. The psoas, pectineus, rectus femoris, and sartorius of the straight leg flex the hip.

6. On the straight leg, the quadriceps contract to straighten the knee.

7. The peroneus longus and brevis muscles turn the ankle of the straight leg slightly outward.

8. The obliques (located toward the side of the abdomen) are activated to increase the turn.

9. The quadratus lumborum and erector spinae arch the back slightly.

Inset: The back portion of the deltoids, the triceps, and the trapezius synergize to deepen the pose.

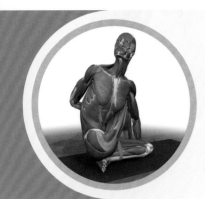

Ardha Matsyendrasana:
Lord of the Fishes Pose

This twisting pose, reminiscent of the salmon twisting as it climbs upstream, uses the energy generated by binding the forward arm to the foot and the other arm (behind the back) to the thigh. We illustrate it here in its intermediate variation, using a belt to reel the back arm into the leg.

Synergizing/Activating

1. The forward arm biceps and brachialis (the muscles at the front of the upper arm) combine with the pectoralis major and activate to deepen the turn of the torso.

2. The outward force of the tensor fascia lata presses the knee against the back of the arm.

3. The posterior deltoid extends the shoulder, pushing the upper arm bone (the humerus) against the knee and opening the chest.

4. The pectoralis and subscapularis muscles work to turn the shoulder inward on the arm behind the back, stretching the infraspinatus and teres minor.

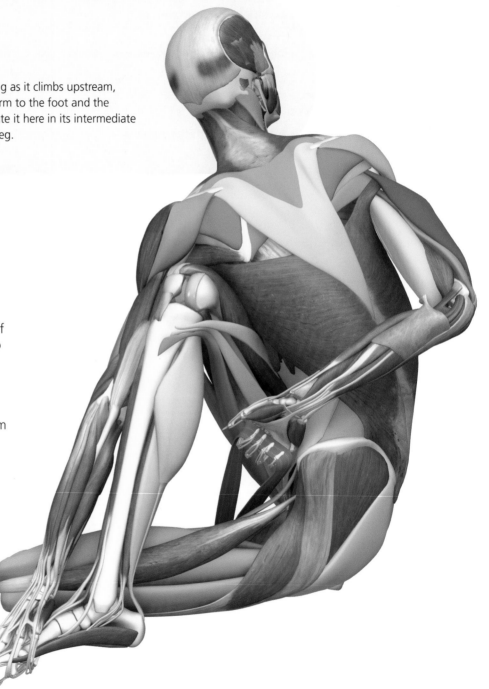

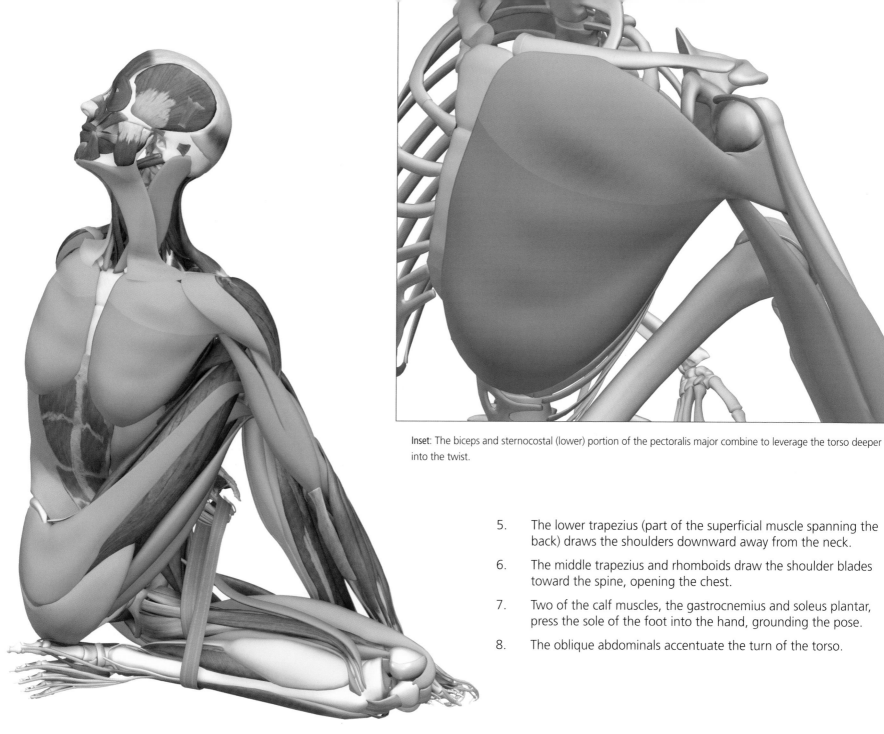

Inset: The biceps and sternocostal (lower) portion of the pectoralis major combine to leverage the torso deeper into the twist.

5.   The lower trapezius (part of the superficial muscle spanning the back) draws the shoulders downward away from the neck.

6.   The middle trapezius and rhomboids draw the shoulder blades toward the spine, opening the chest.

7.   Two of the calf muscles, the gastrocnemius and soleus plantar, press the sole of the foot into the hand, grounding the pose.

8.   The oblique abdominals accentuate the turn of the torso.

Back Bends

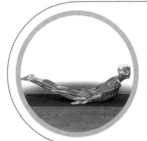

Salabhasana
Locust Pose
Page 132

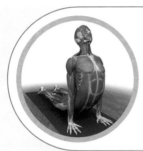

Urdhva Mukha Svanasana
Upward Facing Dog Pose
Page 134

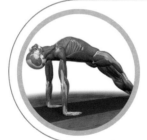

Purvottanasana
Intense Stretch to the East Pose
Page 136

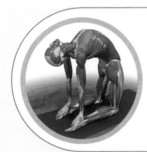

Ustrasana
Camel Pose
Page 138

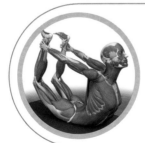

Danurasana
Bow Pose
Page 140

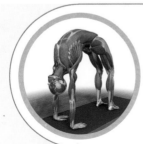

Urdhva Danurasana
Upward Facing Bow Pose
Page 142

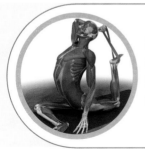

Eka Pada Rajakapotasana I
Pigeon Pose
Page 144

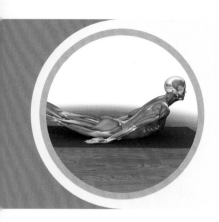

Salabhasana: Locust Pose

Salabhasana strengthens the muscles that arch the back, including the erector spinae along the length of the spine, the quadratus lumborum in the lower back, the lower trapezius spanning the upper back, the gluteus maximus, and the hamstrings. This prepares the body for back bends that create greater extension of the spine, such as Urdhva Danurasana and Ustrasana.

Synergizing/Activating

1. The gluteus maximus extends the hips and tilts the pelvis downward into retroversion.

2. The hamstrings down the back of the thighs extend the hips out and up and lift the knees.

3. The adductors along the inside of the thigh also stretch the hips outward and draw the knees together.

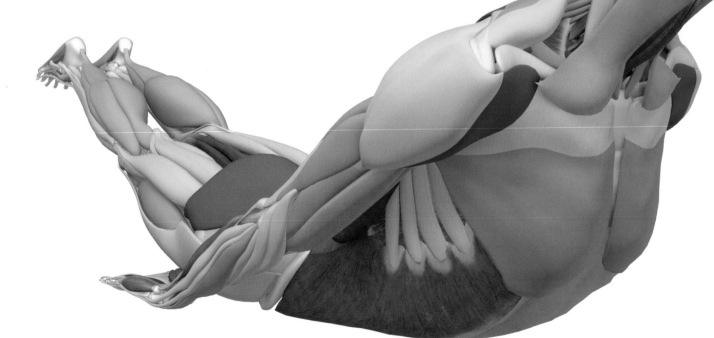

4. The quadriceps straighten the knees.

5. The erector spinae along the length of the spine arch the back.

6. The lower trapezius, spanning the back, draws the shoulders back and down.

7. The posterior deltoids across the back of the shoulders stretch toward the spine.

8. The triceps straighten the elbows.

9. The pectoralis major and minor aid to open the chest.

Inset: The deep hip flexors stretch the psoas, pectineus, and adductor longus.

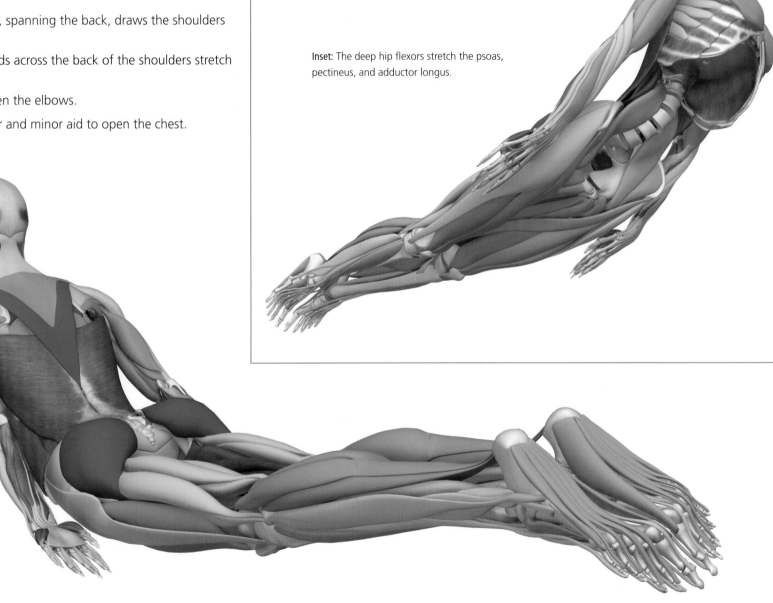

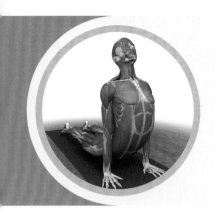

Urdhva Mukha Svanasana:
Upward Facing Dog Pose

This back-bending pose forms part of the Sun Salutations and Vinyasa Flow sequence. It can also be performed alone to strengthen the upper extremities, open the chest, and tone the extensors of the back.

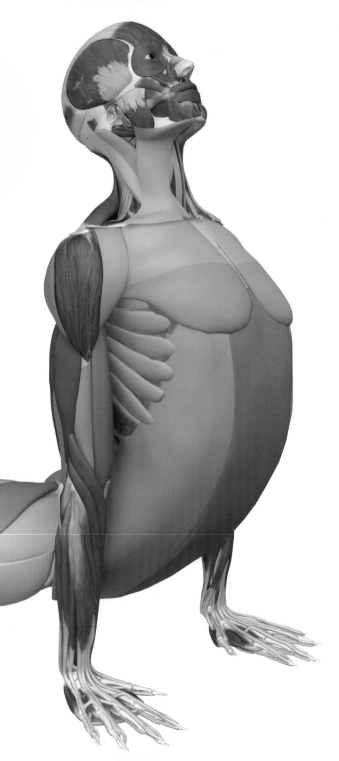

Synergizing/Activating

Shoulders and Arms

1. The triceps muscles at the back of the upper arms straighten the elbows.

2. The back portions of the deltoids activate to draw the shoulders back, extending the upper arm bones, opening the chest, and stretching the upper portion of the pectoralis major.

3. Muscles on the back of the shoulder blades, the infraspinatus and teres minor, turn the shoulders outward to open the chest.

4. The lower portion of the trapezius draws the shoulders down the back and away from the ears.

5. The lower portion of the pectoralis major lifts the chest.

Trunk

1. The erector spinae muscles along the length of the spine arch the back.

2. The glutei in the buttocks combine with the psoas and abdominals to stabilize the pelvis and protect the lower back.

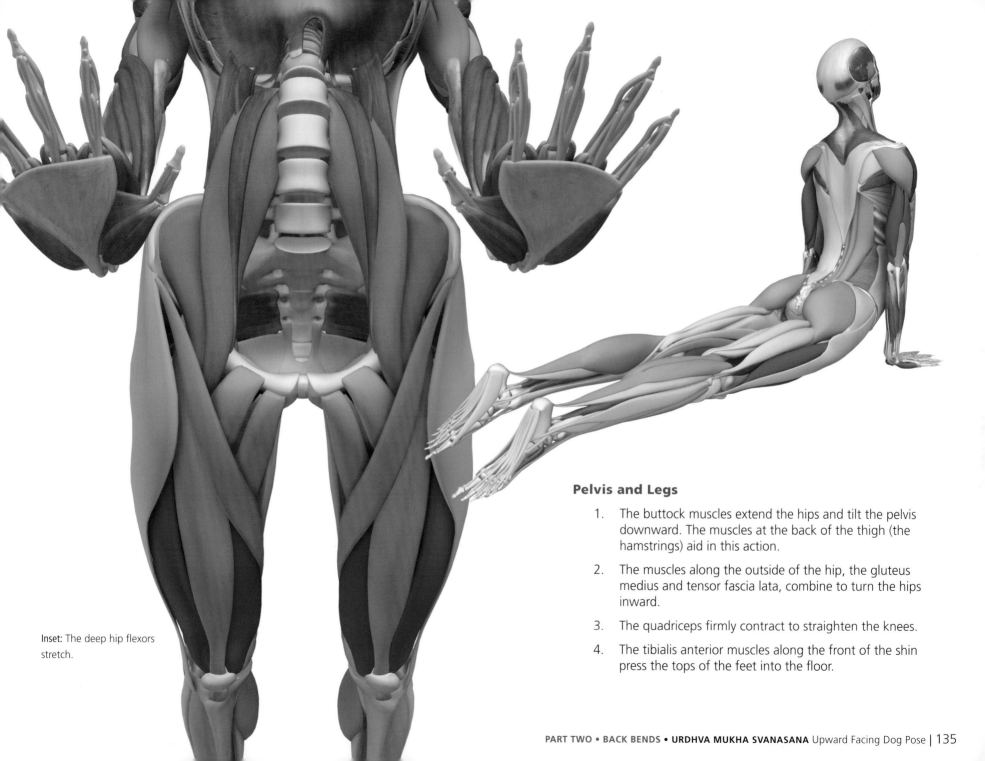

Inset: The deep hip flexors stretch.

Pelvis and Legs

1. The buttock muscles extend the hips and tilt the pelvis downward. The muscles at the back of the thigh (the hamstrings) aid in this action.

2. The muscles along the outside of the hip, the gluteus medius and tensor fascia lata, combine to turn the hips inward.

3. The quadriceps firmly contract to straighten the knees.

4. The tibialis anterior muscles along the front of the shin press the tops of the feet into the floor.

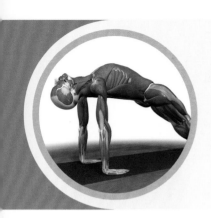

Purvottanasana:
Intense Stretch to the East Pose

Purvottanasana is a back bend in which the shoulders extend, thus the pose is related to Ustrasana. The hips extend less in this pose, focusing the stretch on the shoulders.

Synergizing/Activating

1. The posterior deltoid muscles extend the shoulders back and away from the torso. This creates an intense stretch of the anterior portion of the deltoids in the shoulders, the pectoralis major on the chest, and the biceps muscles on the upper arms.

2. The triceps straighten the elbows, lengthening the biceps.

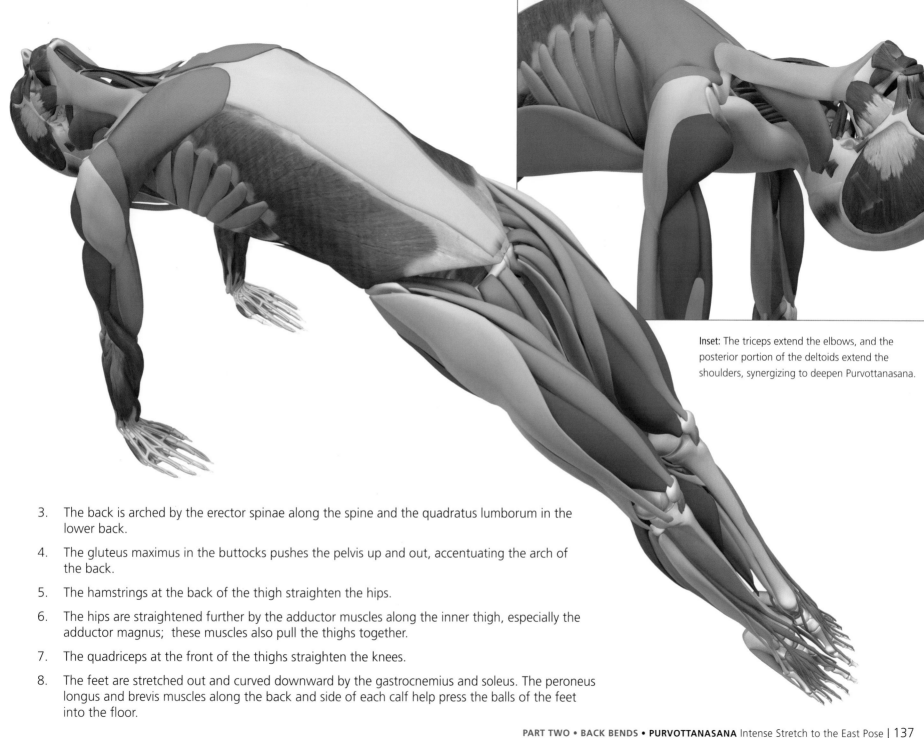

Inset: The triceps extend the elbows, and the posterior portion of the deltoids extend the shoulders, synergizing to deepen Purvottanasana.

3. The back is arched by the erector spinae along the spine and the quadratus lumborum in the lower back.

4. The gluteus maximus in the buttocks pushes the pelvis up and out, accentuating the arch of the back.

5. The hamstrings at the back of the thigh straighten the hips.

6. The hips are straightened further by the adductor muscles along the inner thigh, especially the adductor magnus; these muscles also pull the thighs together.

7. The quadriceps at the front of the thighs straighten the knees.

8. The feet are stretched out and curved downward by the gastrocnemius and soleus. The peroneus longus and brevis muscles along the back and side of each calf help press the balls of the feet into the floor.

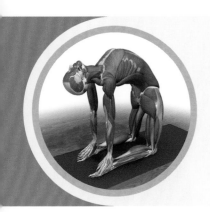

Ustrasana: Camel Pose

Ustrasana is a back bend in which the shoulders extend out behind (as in Purvottanasana). The hands on the feet connect the upper and lower appendicular skeletons (as in Danurasana).

Synergizing/Activating

1. The rhomboids, connecting the spine and the shoulder blades, work with the lower and middle trapezius (spanning the back) to draw the shoulders back and down.

2. The pectoralis minor in the upper chest lifts the rib cage.

3. The posterior deltoids (at the back of the shoulders) extend the upper arm.

4. The triceps, at the back of the upper arms, straighten the elbows.

5. The wrists bend away from the body.

6. The gluteus maximus in the buttocks and the hamstrings down the back of the thigh straighten the hips.

7. The adductors in the inner thigh press the hips straighter and draw the thigh bones toward the body.

8. The tensor fascia lata (down the outside of the hips) and the gluteus medius in the buttocks turn the thigh bones inward. This action counters the turning out of the thighs created by the gluteus maximus.

9. The quadriceps (down the front of the thighs) partially straighten the knees to bring the thigh bones to a right angle to the floor.

10. The gastrocnemius and soleus, the calf muscles, bend the ankles away from the shins.

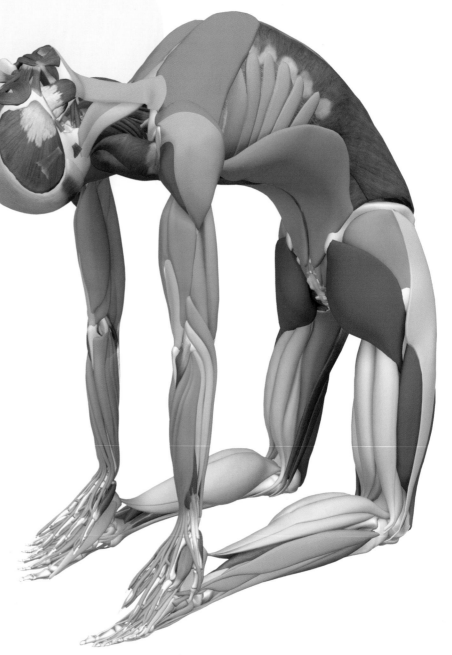

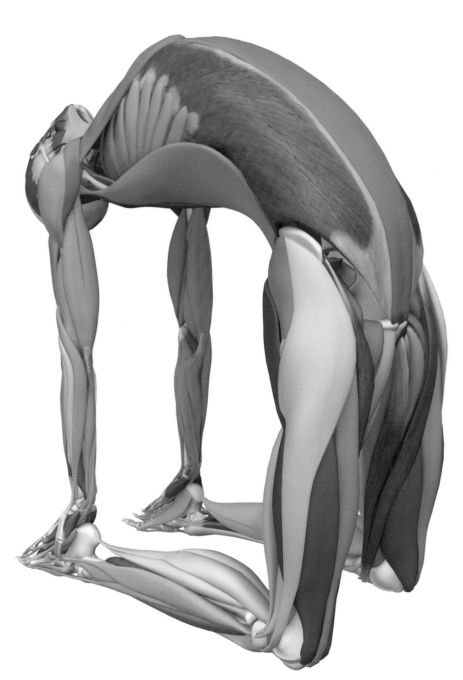

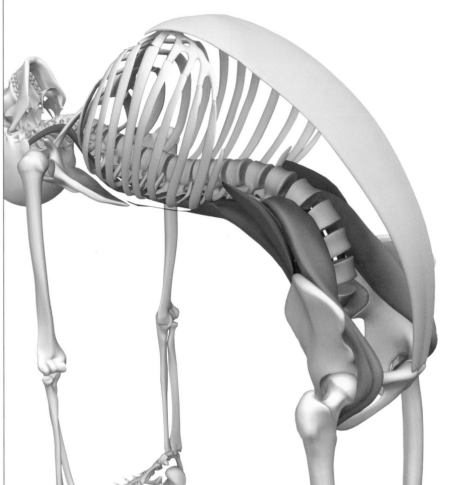

Inset: The psoas and quadratus lumborum surround the lumbar spine, protecting it. The rectus abdominis lightly contracts. This creates the "abdominal airbag effect," pressing the abdominal organs against the spine, further protecting it.

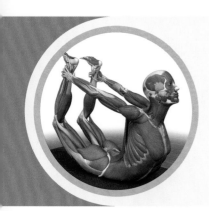

Danurasana: Bow Pose

Here the torso and legs form the body of a bow and the arms form the string. Contracting the muscles on the back of the body slackens the string. Keeping the muscles along the front of the body active tightens the bow. Further bending the elbows draws the string and bends the bow.

Synergizing/Activating

1. The posterior deltoids (muscles at the back of the shoulders) and the triceps at the back of the upper arm extend the elbows, allowing the hands to grip the ankles. This attaches the string of the bow. The biceps bend the elbows, tightening the string, and thus draw the bow.

2. The hamstrings (along the back of the thigh) bend the knees, bringing the ankles to the hands.

3. The tibialis anterior muscles on the front of the shins bend the ankles toward the shins; along the outside of the calf, the peroneus longus and brevis turn the ankle slightly outward. These actions "lock" the attachment of the hands to the ankles.

4. The lower trapezius (spanning the back) and the rhomboids (between the shoulder blades and the spine) draw the shoulders back and down, opening the chest.

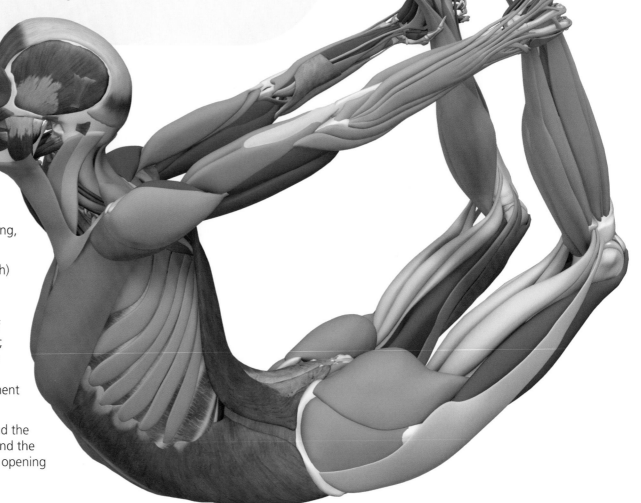

Inset: The hip flexors and rectus abdominis stretch.

5. The quadriceps straighten the knees, tightening the bow.

6. The buttocks muscle works to extend the hips.

7. The erector spinae (running the length of the spine) and the quadratus lumborum in the small of the back arch the back.

8. Gently activating the rectus abdominis on the front of the body creates the "abdominal airbag" effect by compressing the abdominal organs against the spine. At the same time, this softens the arching of the lumbar spine.

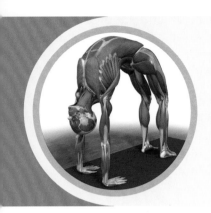

Urdhva Danurasana: Upward Facing Bow Pose

Urdhva Danurasana creates a back bend with the shoulders fully flexed over the head. This differs from Danurasana (bow pose), in which the shoulders extend back away from the torso. This means that other muscle groups are working and stretching, especially around the shoulders.

Synergizing/Activating

Shoulders and Arms

1. The triceps at the back of the upper arms straighten the elbows. Contracting the long head of these upper arm muscles turns the tail of the shoulder blade outwards and helps stabilize the head of the upper arm bone (the humerus) in the socket of the shoulder joint.

2. The anterior deltoids bend the shoulders back toward the floor.

3. The infraspinatus and teres minor muscles (across the shoulder blades and back of the shoulders) turn the shoulders outward.

4. The upper trapezius (that spans the back) elevates the shoulder girdle.

5. The middle trapezius and the rhomboids, connected to the spine and the shoulder blades, draw the shoulder blades toward the midline.

6. The lower trapezius draws the shoulders away from the neck.

7. The wrist extensors along the forearms bend the wrists toward the forearm.

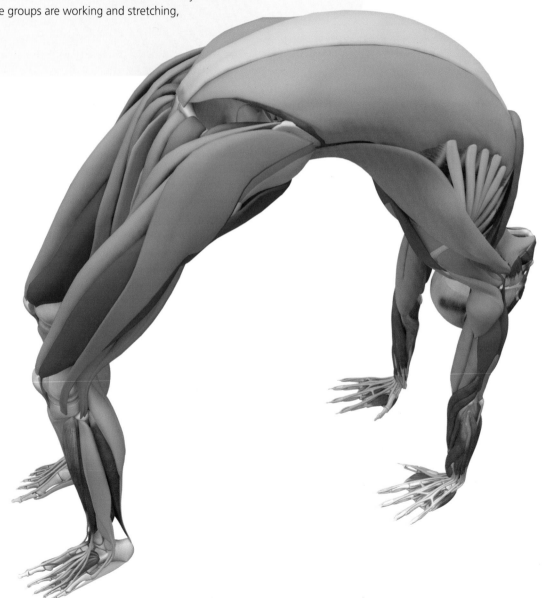

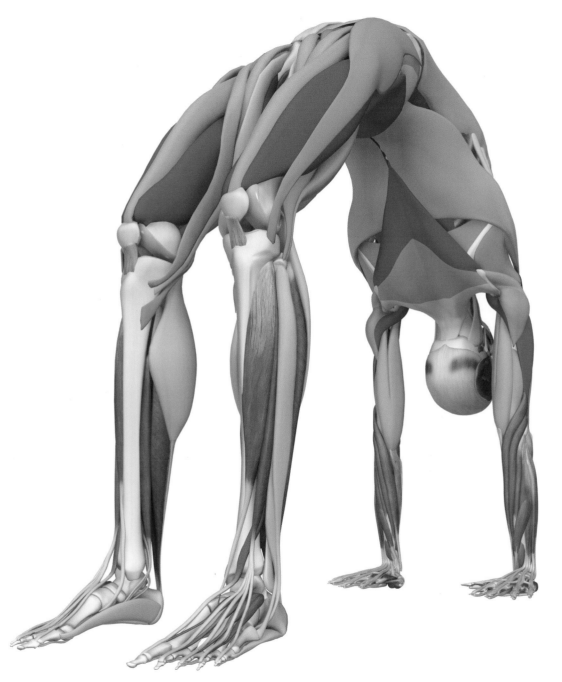

Trunk

1. The erector spinae, which flow the length of the spine, arch the back.

2. The quadratus lumborum muscles in the lower back work with the psoas (high at the front of the thigh) to stabilize the lower back.

3. The rectus abdominis, which flows from the chest to the pubic bone, contracts lightly to obtain the "abdominal airbag" effect, adding more protection for the lower back.

Pelvis and Legs

1. The gluteus maximus in the buttocks and the hamstrings (down the back of the thigh) extend the hips.

2. The tensor fascia lata (along the outside of the hip) and the gluteus medius (deep in the buttocks) turn the hips and the thigh bones inward.

3. The adductors on the inner thigh straighten the thigh bones, drawing them toward the body.

4. The quadriceps (down the front of the thighs) straighten the knees.

5. The peronei (along the outside of the calf) turn the ankles slightly outward.

6. The gastrocnemius and soleus (muscles in the calf) press the feet down, grounding the pose.

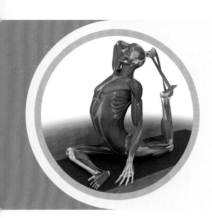

Eka Pada Rajakapotasana I: Pigeon Pose

This is an advanced back bend. We illustrate an intermediate variation using a belt to aid in grasping the foot. Pay particular attention to the chest in this pose. Pigeon helps to lift and open the chest by activating the pectoralis minor muscles, located at the upper part of the chest, and the rhomboid muscles, which connect the spine to the shoulder blades.

Synergizing/Activating

1. The forward leg is rotated outward by the psoas, which is located high at the front of the thigh; by the sartorius, which is attached to the pelvis and thigh bone; and by the deep external rotators in the thigh, which have a turning capacity.

2. The tensor fascia lata and gluteus medius of the forward leg lengthen as the hip turns outward.

3. The thigh bone is moved away from the midline by the sartorius and the gluteus medius in the buttocks.

4. The hamstrings of the forward leg bend the knee.

5. The gluteus maximus in the buttocks of the back leg presses the hip forward, tilts the pelvis downward, and extends the thigh bone.

6. The gluteus medius works with the tensor fascia lata along the side of the back hip to turn the hip inward.

7. The hamstrings bend the back knee and further extend the hip.

8. The tibialis anterior and peronei along the edge of the shin and the calf bend and slightly turn the ankle outward. These actions create a place to grip the foot and connect the upper and lower extremities.

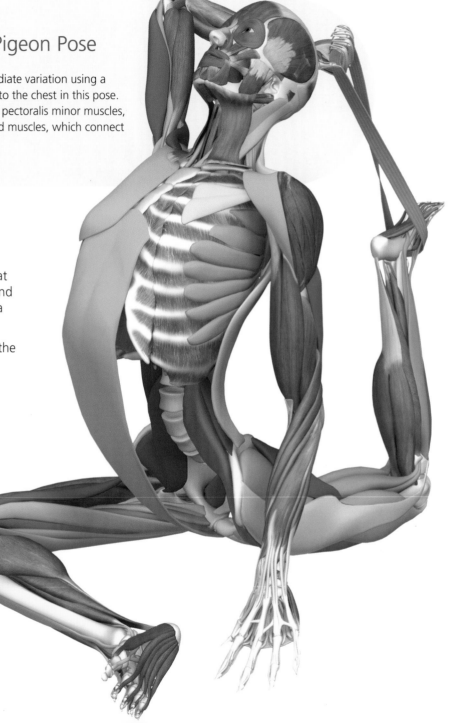

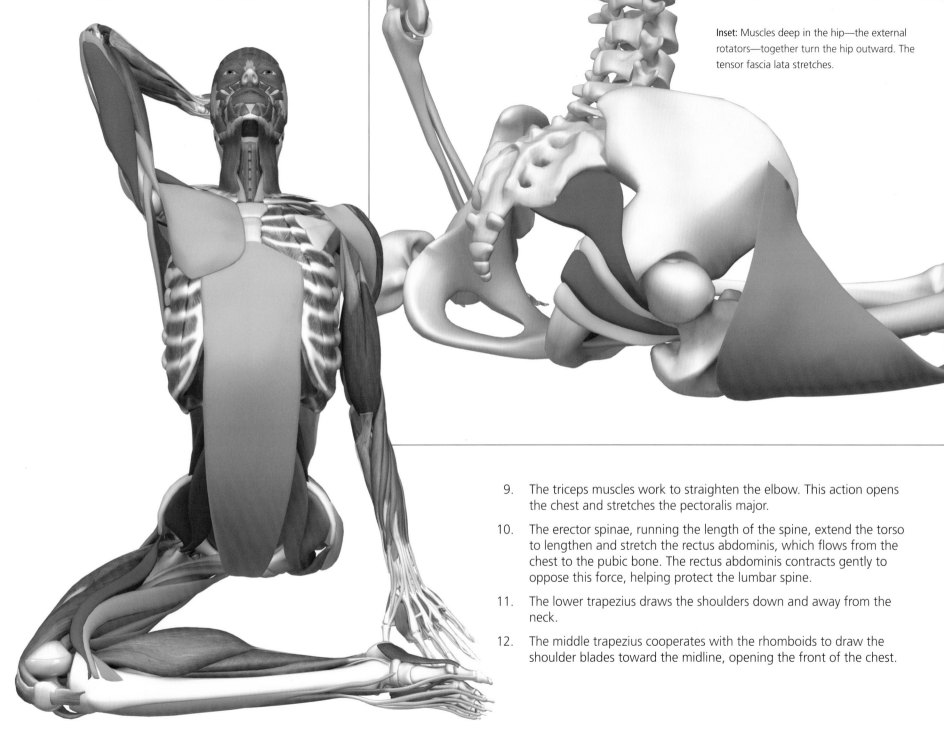

Inset: Muscles deep in the hip—the external rotators—together turn the hip outward. The tensor fascia lata stretches.

9. The triceps muscles work to straighten the elbow. This action opens the chest and stretches the pectoralis major.

10. The erector spinae, running the length of the spine, extend the torso to lengthen and stretch the rectus abdominis, which flows from the chest to the pubic bone. The rectus abdominis contracts gently to oppose this force, helping protect the lumbar spine.

11. The lower trapezius draws the shoulders down and away from the neck.

12. The middle trapezius cooperates with the rhomboids to draw the shoulder blades toward the midline, opening the front of the chest.

Arm Balances

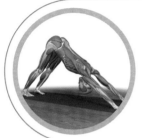

Adho Mukha Svanasana
Downward Facing Dog
Page 148

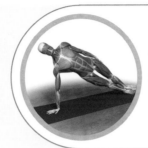

Vasisthasana
Sage Pose
Page 150

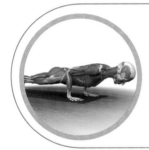

Chataranga Dandasana
Four Limb Staff Pose
Page 152

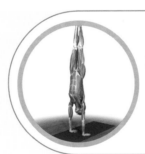

Adho Mukha Vrksasana
Full Arm Balance
Page 154

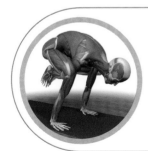

Bakasana
Crow Pose
Page 156

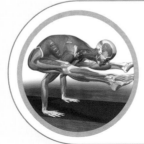

Titibasana
Insect Pose
Page 160

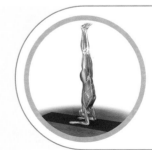

Pincha Mayurasana
Feather of the Peacock Pose
Page 162

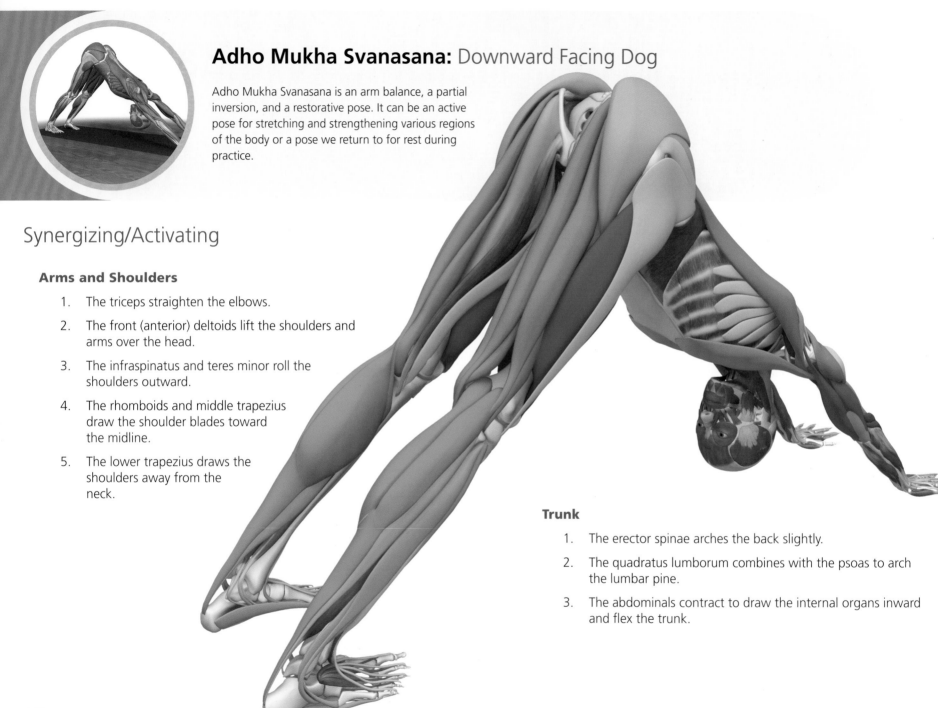

Adho Mukha Svanasana: Downward Facing Dog

Adho Mukha Svanasana is an arm balance, a partial inversion, and a restorative pose. It can be an active pose for stretching and strengthening various regions of the body or a pose we return to for rest during practice.

Synergizing/Activating

Arms and Shoulders

1. The triceps straighten the elbows.

2. The front (anterior) deltoids lift the shoulders and arms over the head.

3. The infraspinatus and teres minor roll the shoulders outward.

4. The rhomboids and middle trapezius draw the shoulder blades toward the midline.

5. The lower trapezius draws the shoulders away from the neck.

Trunk

1. The erector spinae arches the back slightly.

2. The quadratus lumborum combines with the psoas to arch the lumbar pine.

3. The abdominals contract to draw the internal organs inward and flex the trunk.

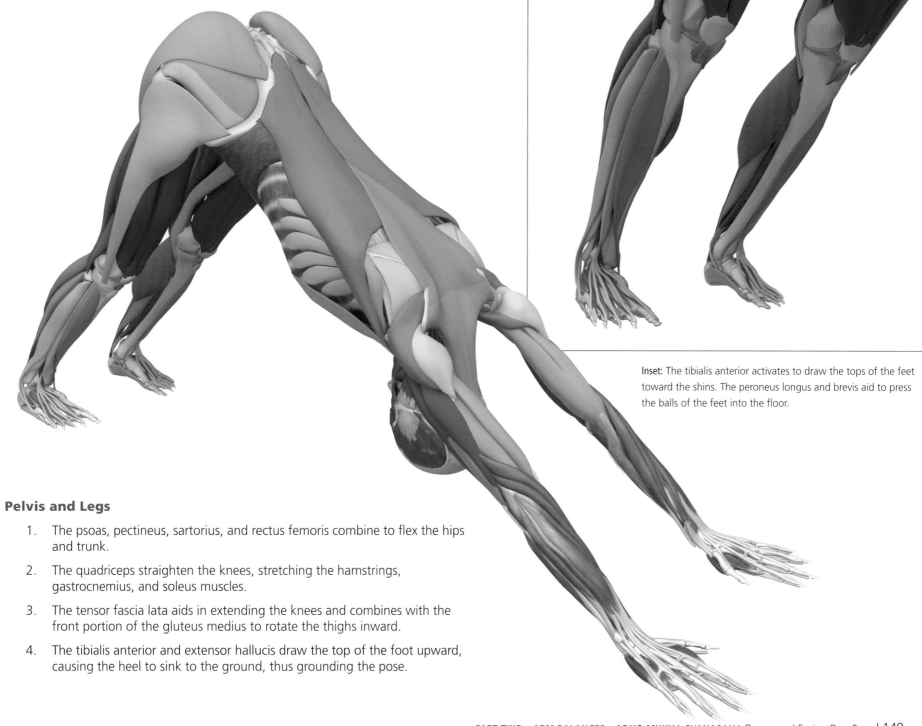

Inset: The tibialis anterior activates to draw the tops of the feet toward the shins. The peroneus longus and brevis aid to press the balls of the feet into the floor.

Pelvis and Legs

1. The psoas, pectineus, sartorius, and rectus femoris combine to flex the hips and trunk.

2. The quadriceps straighten the knees, stretching the hamstrings, gastrocnemius, and soleus muscles.

3. The tensor fascia lata aids in extending the knees and combines with the front portion of the gluteus medius to rotate the thighs inward.

4. The tibialis anterior and extensor hallucis draw the top of the foot upward, causing the heel to sink to the ground, thus grounding the pose.

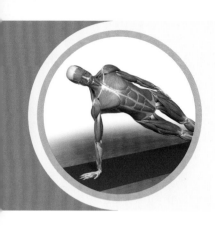

Vasisthasana: Sage Pose

Vasisthasana is named for the sage Vasistha. It is an arm balance on one side and is useful for isolating and strengthening the deep and superficial shoulder muscles, including those of the rotator cuff. It also strengthens the muscular stabilizers of the wrist and elbow and teaches balance.

Synergizing/Activating

Shoulders and Arms

1. The triceps of the balancing arm firmly contract to straighten the elbow, lengthening the biceps.

2. The lateral (middle) portion of the deltoids activate to draw the arm away from the side of the body. The front and back portions of the deltoids refine this action.

3. The supraspinatus muscle deep in the shoulder aids to draw the arm away from the side, with the infraspinatus and teres minor turning the arm outward and stabilizing the head of the humerus in the shoulder socket.

4. The upper (sternoclavicular) portion of the pectoralis major muscle combines with the trapezius to stabilize the upper arm and shoulder girdle.

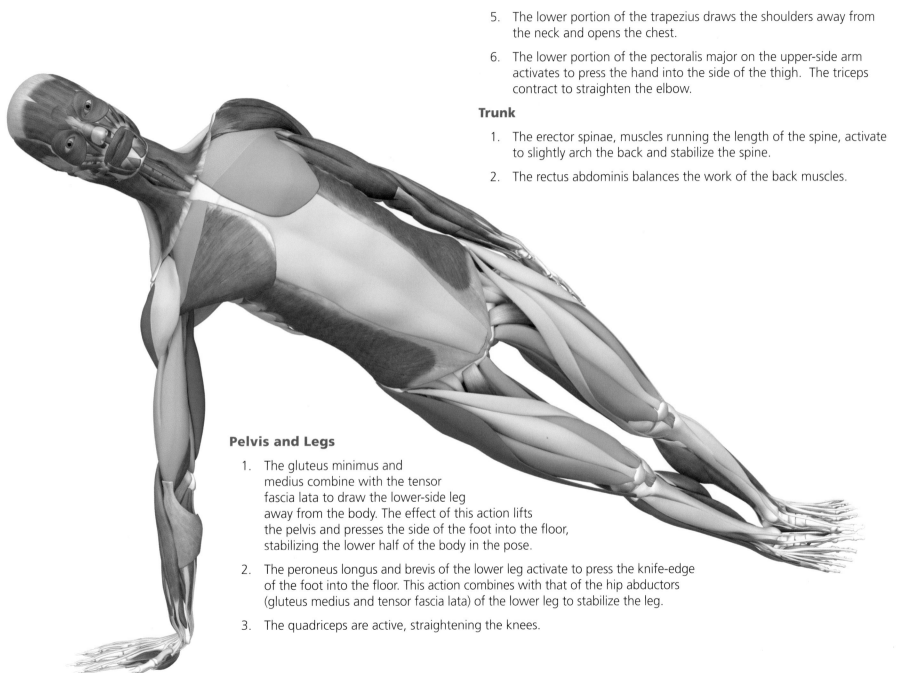

5. The lower portion of the trapezius draws the shoulders away from the neck and opens the chest.

6. The lower portion of the pectoralis major on the upper-side arm activates to press the hand into the side of the thigh. The triceps contract to straighten the elbow.

Trunk

1. The erector spinae, muscles running the length of the spine, activate to slightly arch the back and stabilize the spine.

2. The rectus abdominis balances the work of the back muscles.

Pelvis and Legs

1. The gluteus minimus and medius combine with the tensor fascia lata to draw the lower-side leg away from the body. The effect of this action lifts the pelvis and presses the side of the foot into the floor, stabilizing the lower half of the body in the pose.

2. The peroneus longus and brevis of the lower leg activate to press the knife-edge of the foot into the floor. This action combines with that of the hip abductors (gluteus medius and tensor fascia lata) of the lower leg to stabilize the leg.

3. The quadriceps are active, straightening the knees.

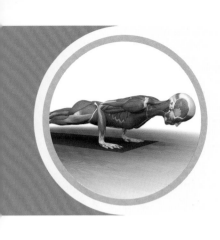

Chataranga Dandasana: Four Limb Staff Pose

Many Yoga systems use this pose to transition from Uttanasana to Upward Facing Dog pose during the Sun Salutations or in Vinyasa Flow sequences. You can also practice it as a stand alone posture, holding it for a longer period to strengthen a number of core muscles and to activate the core Bandhas.

Synergizing/Activating

1. Located on both sides of the rib cage, the serratus anterior muscles reach to the center-line border of the inside of the shoulder blades, tethering them and preventing them from "winging" upward.

2. The rhomboids connect the shoulder blades to the spine and work with the midsection of the trapezius to draw the shoulder blades toward the midline. This action combines with that of the serratus anterior to stabilize the shoulder blades and the entire shoulder.

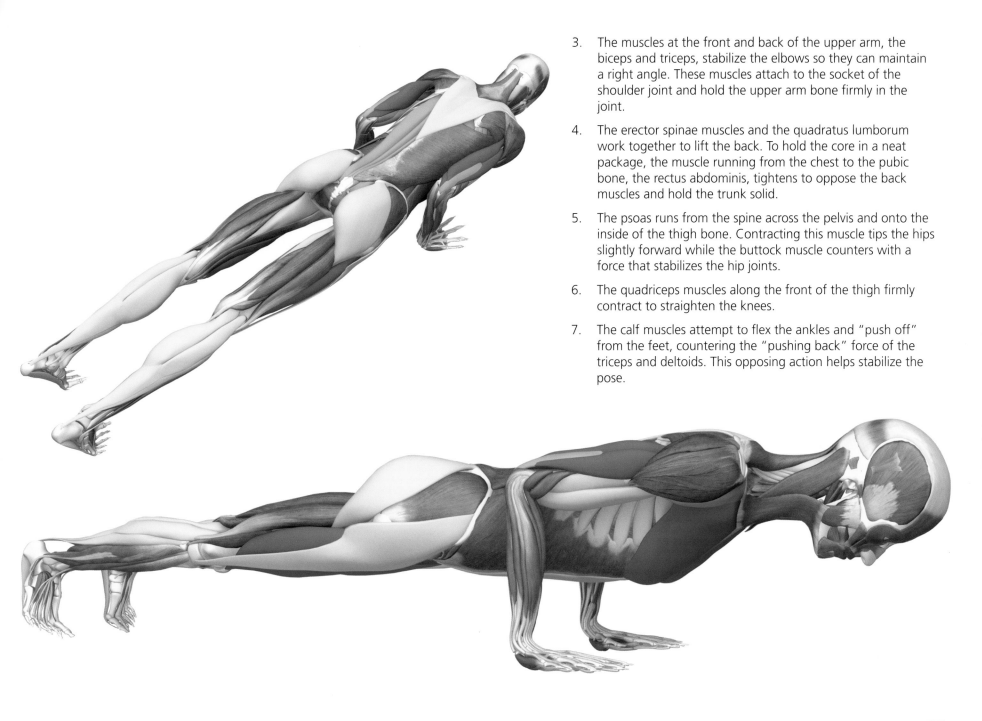

3. The muscles at the front and back of the upper arm, the biceps and triceps, stabilize the elbows so they can maintain a right angle. These muscles attach to the socket of the shoulder joint and hold the upper arm bone firmly in the joint.

4. The erector spinae muscles and the quadratus lumborum work together to lift the back. To hold the core in a neat package, the muscle running from the chest to the pubic bone, the rectus abdominis, tightens to oppose the back muscles and hold the trunk solid.

5. The psoas runs from the spine across the pelvis and onto the inside of the thigh bone. Contracting this muscle tips the hips slightly forward while the buttock muscle counters with a force that stabilizes the hip joints.

6. The quadriceps muscles along the front of the thigh firmly contract to straighten the knees.

7. The calf muscles attempt to flex the ankles and "push off" from the feet, countering the "pushing back" force of the triceps and deltoids. This opposing action helps stabilize the pose.

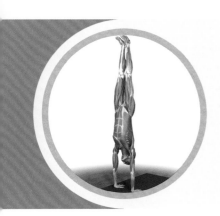

Adho Mukha Vrksasana: Full Arm Balance

Practicing arm balances, such as Adho Mukha Vrksasana, strengthens the core muscles of the shoulder girdle and arms. This increases the stability of the shoulder joint. This pose is also a dynamic type of inversion with beneficial effects on the cardiovascular and nervous system.

Synergizing/Activating

1. The triceps extend the elbows, aligning the bones of the upper arms and forearms.

2. The biceps are active, balancing the force of the triceps and preventing hyperextension of the elbows.

3. The long heads of the triceps and biceps cross the shoulder joint. Contracting these muscles stabilizes the humerus in the glenoid (socket) of the shoulder joint.

4. The infraspinatus and teres minor externally rotate the humerus to avoid impingement of the humerus on the acromion process.

5. The anterior deltoids flex the shoulders over the head.

6. The lower trapezius draws the shoulders away from the cervical spine, freeing the neck.

7. The psoas and gluteus maximus create opposing forces to stabilize the hips and balance the pelvis.

8. The adductor group draws the thighs toward the midline.

9. The quadriceps extend the knees.

10. The peroneus longus and brevis evert the ankles and open the soles of the feet.

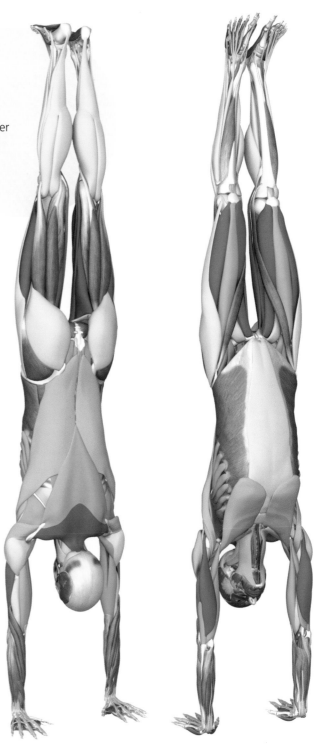

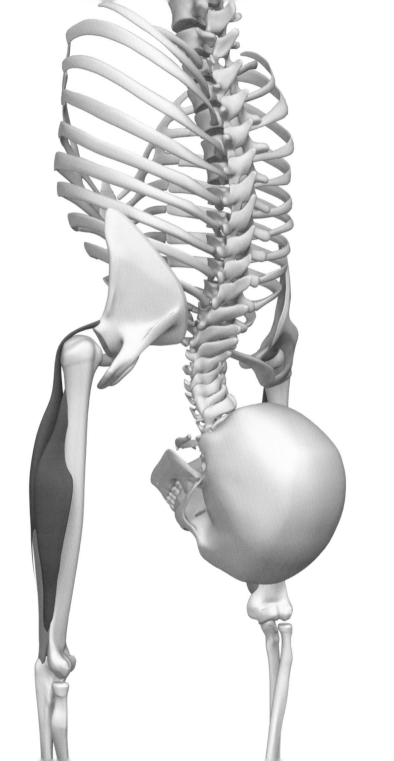

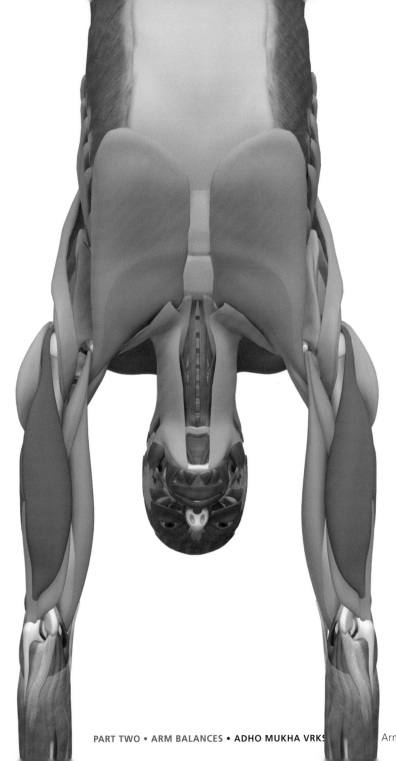

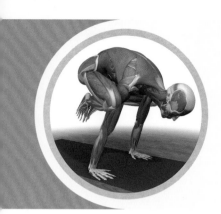

Bakasana: Crow Pose

This balancing pose resembles a crow perching on a tree. It connects the upper and lower extremities to improve balance and stability.

Synergizing/Activating

1. The serratus anterior, the muscle connecting the side of the rib cage to the shoulder blade, draws the shoulder blades forward, stretching both the middle trapezius and the rhomboids.

2. The pectoralis major combines with the anterior deltoids to stabilize the shoulders.

3. The lower trapezius, which spans the back, presses down on the shoulder blades.

4. The infraspinatus and teres minor turn the humerus (the upper arm bone) outward to refine shoulder stability.

5. The triceps straighten the elbows to mimic the crow's legs.

6. The hamstrings bend the knees.

7. The adductor muscle group in the inner thighs squeezes the knees into the upper arms, like folded wings, linking the upper and lower extremities.

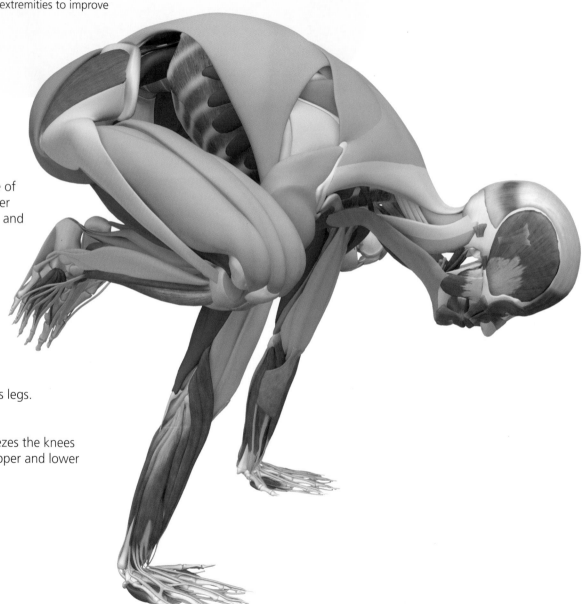

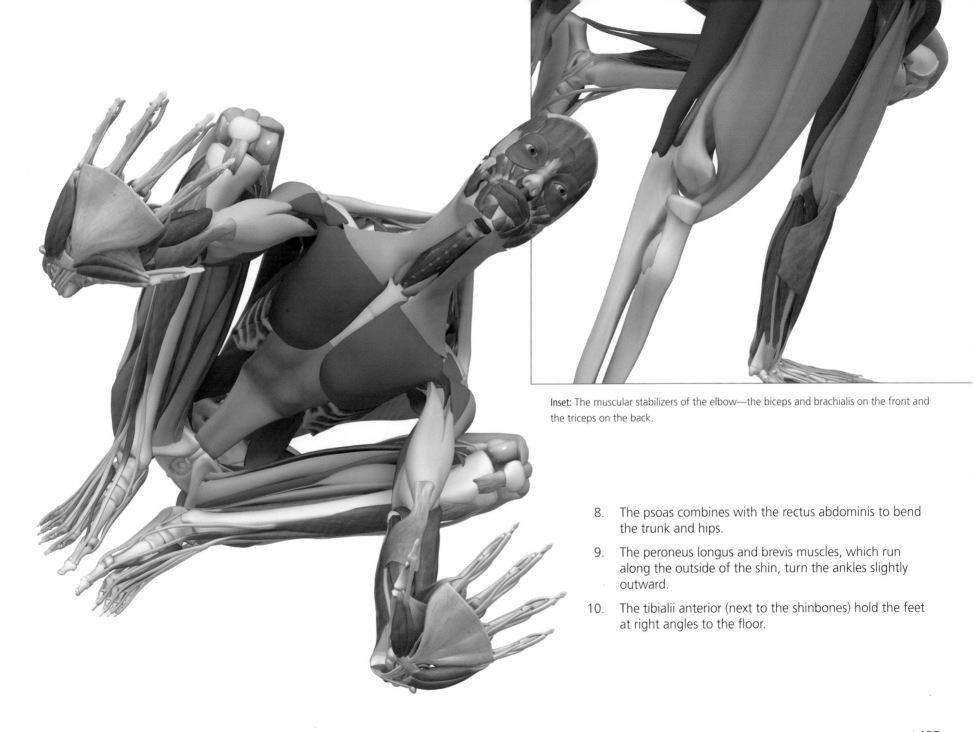

Inset: The muscular stabilizers of the elbow—the biceps and brachialis on the front and the triceps on the back.

8. The psoas combines with the rectus abdominis to bend the trunk and hips.

9. The peroneus longus and brevis muscles, which run along the outside of the shin, turn the ankles slightly outward.

10. The tibialii anterior (next to the shinbones) hold the feet at right angles to the floor.

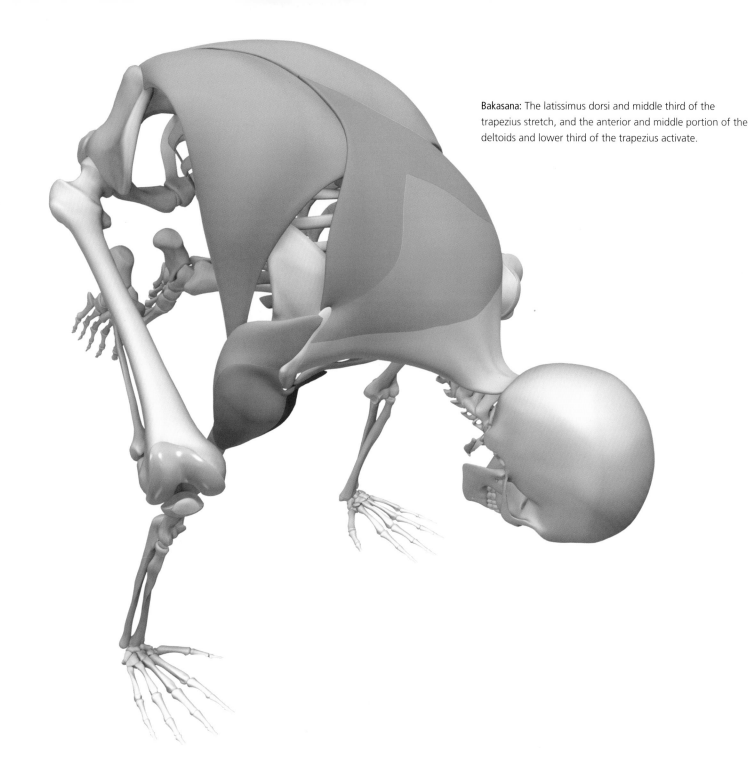

Bakasana: The latissimus dorsi and middle third of the trapezius stretch, and the anterior and middle portion of the deltoids and lower third of the trapezius activate.

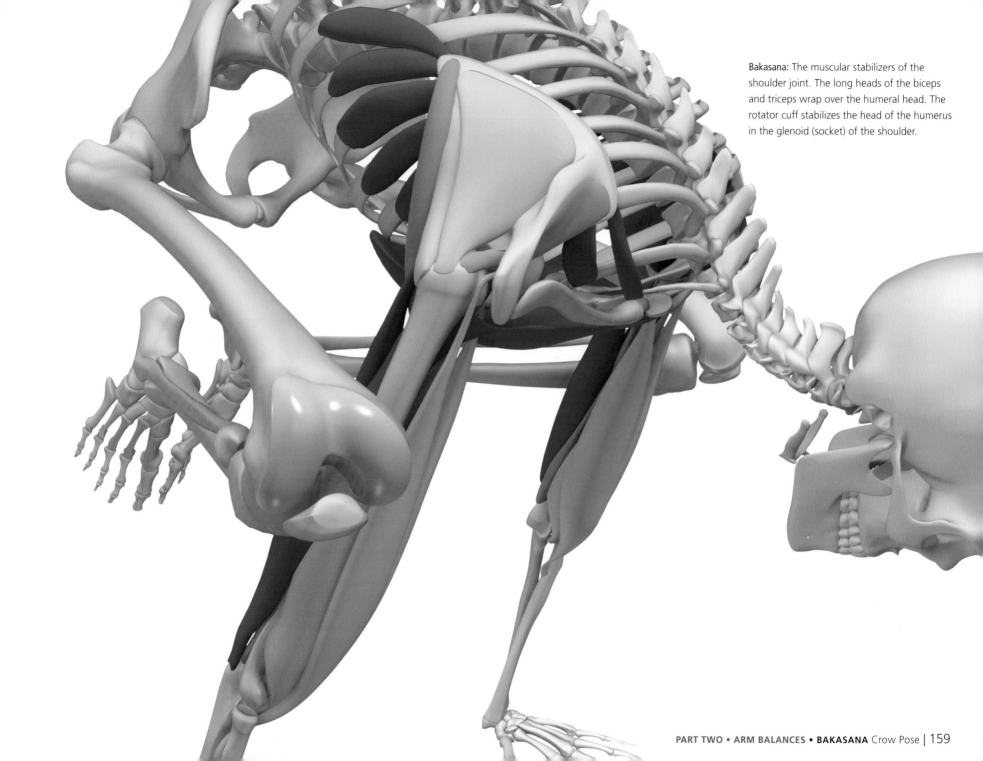

Bakasana: The muscular stabilizers of the shoulder joint. The long heads of the biceps and triceps wrap over the humeral head. The rotator cuff stabilizes the head of the humerus in the glenoid (socket) of the shoulder.

Titibasana: Insect Pose

This pose is similar to Bakasana. It strengthens the upper body and links the upper and lower appendicular skeletons to create stability. Titibasana also strengthens the quadriceps and psoas muscles, stretching the back of the body in the process. It is related to Kurmasana.

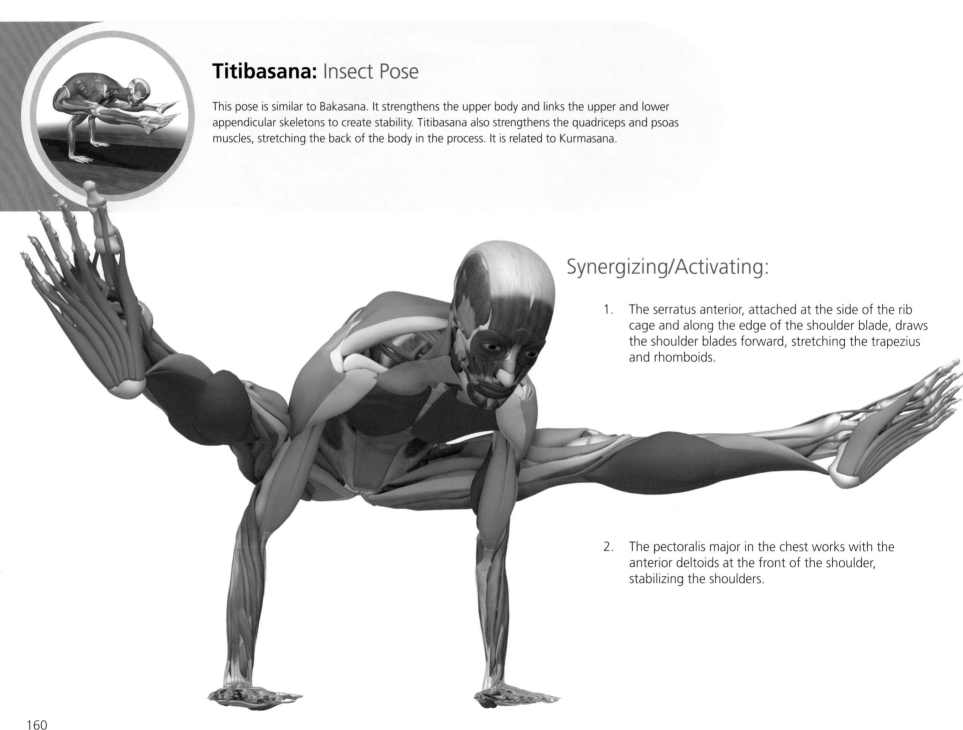

Synergizing/Activating:

1. The serratus anterior, attached at the side of the rib cage and along the edge of the shoulder blade, draws the shoulder blades forward, stretching the trapezius and rhomboids.

2. The pectoralis major in the chest works with the anterior deltoids at the front of the shoulder, stabilizing the shoulders.

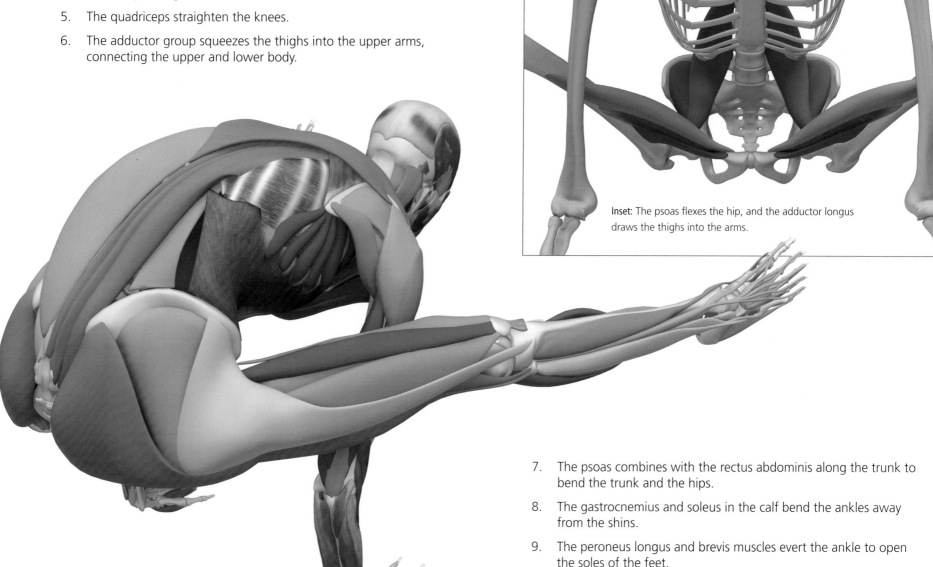

3. The infraspinatus and teres minor turn the humerus (upper arm bone) outward to increase shoulder stability.

4. The triceps straighten the elbows.

5. The quadriceps straighten the knees.

6. The adductor group squeezes the thighs into the upper arms, connecting the upper and lower body.

Inset: The psoas flexes the hip, and the adductor longus draws the thighs into the arms.

7. The psoas combines with the rectus abdominis along the trunk to bend the trunk and the hips.

8. The gastrocnemius and soleus in the calf bend the ankles away from the shins.

9. The peroneus longus and brevis muscles evert the ankle to open the soles of the feet.

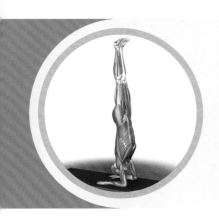

Pincha Mayurasana:
Feather of the Peacock Pose

Pincha Mayurasana is a balancing pose in which the body forms the slight arch of a feather. Proper alignment of the shoulders and hips leads to a feeling of lightness and ease in the pose. The deep and superficial shoulder muscles are strengthened as one balances and aligns the shoulder and hip girdles.

Synergizing/Activating:

Shoulders and Arms

1. The infraspinatus and teres minor are active, turning the shoulders outward and lengthening the subscapularis muscle.

2. The triceps activate to press the forearms down. Extending the elbows assists the wrist flexors to press the palms into the floor.

3. The biceps are active, counterbalancing the triceps to assist in stabilizing the elbows and shoulders.

4. The trapezius and rhomboids draw the shoulder blades toward the midline, opening the chest. The lower third of the trapezius draws the shoulders away from the neck, freeing the cervical spine to extend.

5. The front and middle portions of the deltoids activate to lift the body.

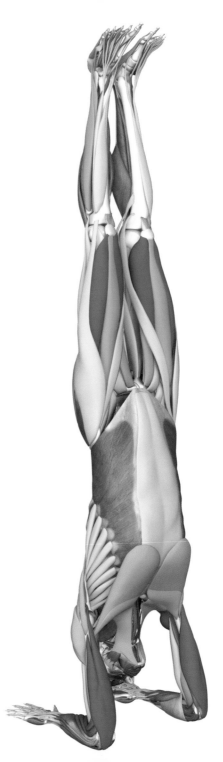

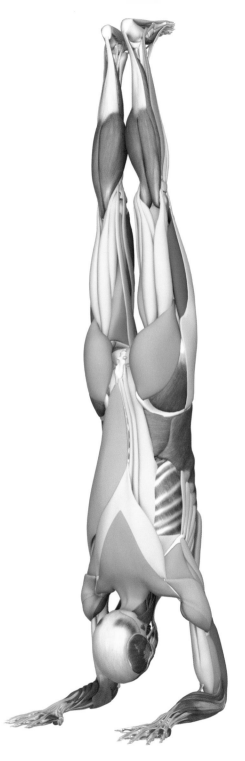

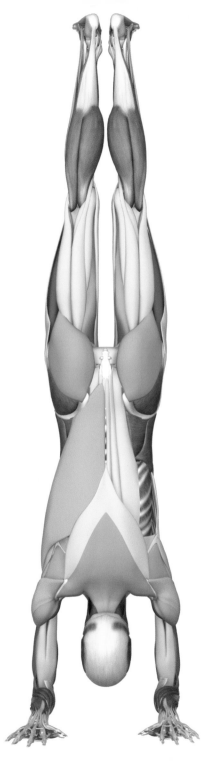

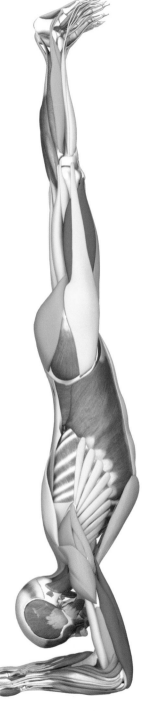

Trunk

1. The erector spinae, flowing the length of the spine, slightly arch the back like a feather. The quadratus lumborum stabilizes the lower back.

2. The rectus abdominis gently activates to counterbalance the arch.

Pelvis and Legs

1. The psoas and gluteals are active, stabilizing the pelvis and preventing sway of the body.

2. The adductor group draws the legs together.

3. The quadriceps straighten the knees.

Inversions

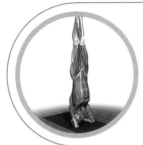

Sirsasana
Headstand
Page 166

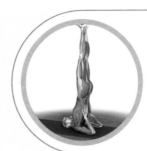

Sarvangasana
Shoulder Stand
Page 170

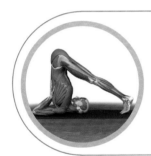

Halasana
Plow Pose
Page 174

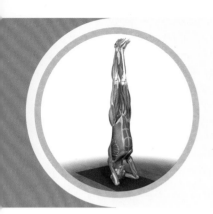

Sirsasana: Headstand

Headstand is a type of restorative pose. It is typically performed near the end of a practice session. Inverting the body stimulates control mechanisms in the heart and the arteries that monitor and adjust blood pressure. Inversions may also positively affect the flow of cerebrospinal fluid in the spinal cord and the brain.

Learn this pose only under the guidance of an experienced teacher. It should not be attempted by anyone who has spinal injuries or other conditions affecting the spine, especially the neck. Practitioners who do have such conditions should work with other poses that invert the body, but do not place undue pressure on the cervical spine. Supported Setu Bandha is an example of such a pose.

Synergizing/Activating

Shoulders and Arms

1. The triceps are active, stabilizing the forearms on the floor.

2. The biceps counteract the action of the triceps. The long heads of both muscles cross the shoulder joint and attach to the joint socket at the top and bottom. Contracting these muscles holds the head of the arm bone firmly in the joint socket.

3. The anterior deltoids draw the shoulders over the head.

4. The lower trapezius draws the shoulders away from the neck, freeing the cervical spine.

5. The infraspinatus and teres minor muscles that join the shoulder blades to the upper arm bone (the humerus) turn its head into the socket, stabilizing it.

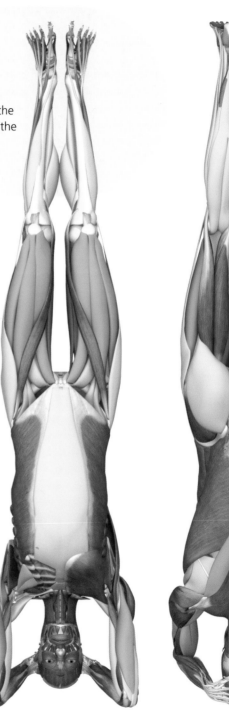

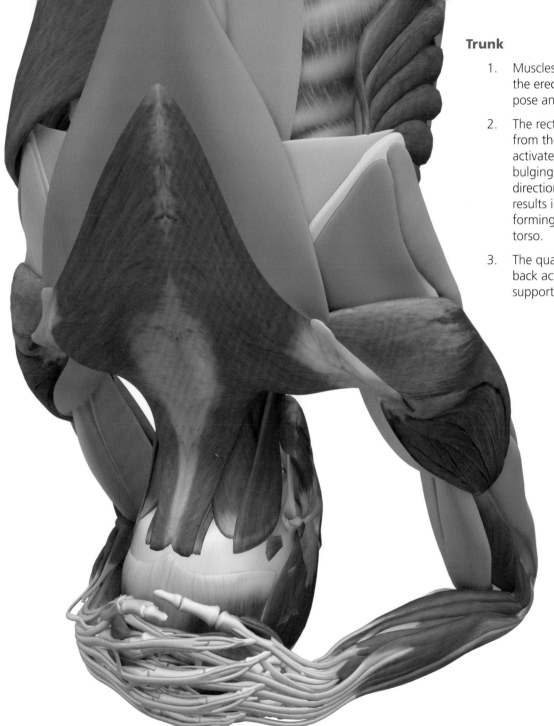

Trunk

1. Muscles running the length of the spine, the erector spinae, lift the back into the pose and remain active to stabilize it.

2. The rectus abdominis muscle, running from the chest to the pubic bone, activates to prevent the rib cage from bulging out. It works in an opposite direction to the erector spinae, which results in the two muscle groups forming a supportive sheath around the torso.

3. The quadratus lumborum in the lower back acts in concert with the psoas to support the lower back.

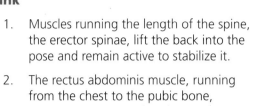
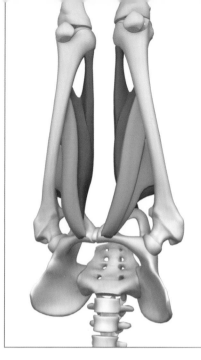

Inset: The adductor group draws the legs together to stabilize the lower body in the inversion.

Pelvis and Legs

1. The gluteus maximus in the buttocks extends the hips. Opposing this at the front, the psoas balances the pelvis so that it is tipped neither forward nor backward, but is straight up and down like an upside down bowl.

2. The tensor fascia lata along the outside of the hip works with the gluteus medius deep in the buttocks to turn the hips inward and keep the legs from splaying. This counteracts the gluteus maximus in turning the hips outward.

3. The adductor group draws the thighs together.

4. The quadriceps straighten the knees.

5. The tibialis anterior muscle on the front of the shin bends the ankles.

6. The peronei muscles along the outside of the lower leg turn the feet slightly outward.

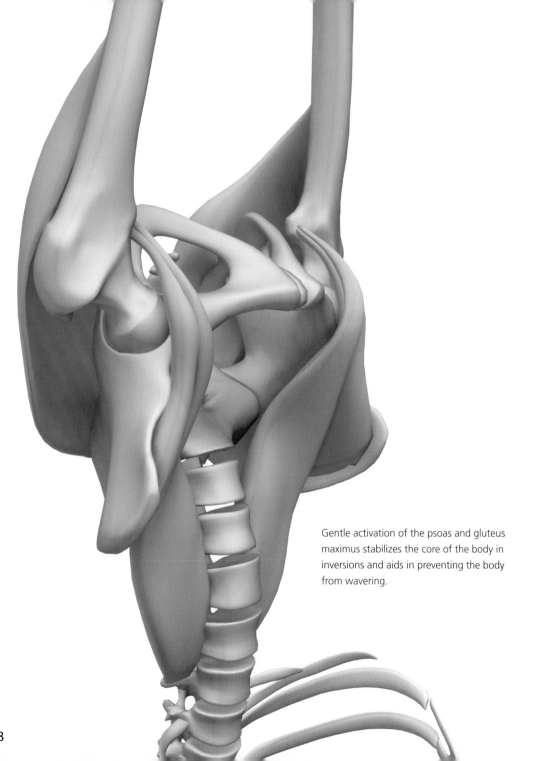

Gentle activation of the psoas and gluteus maximus stabilizes the core of the body in inversions and aids in preventing the body from wavering.

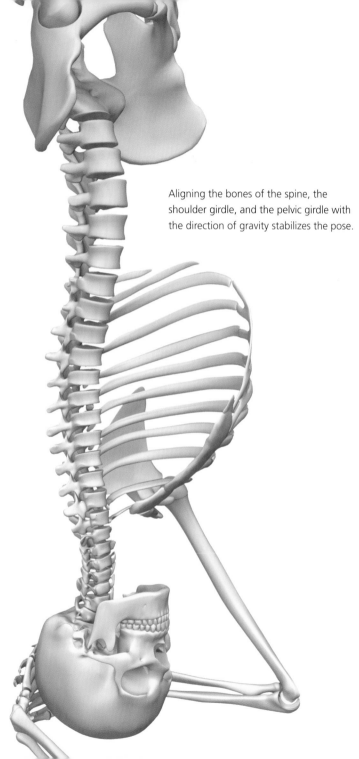

Aligning the bones of the spine, the shoulder girdle, and the pelvic girdle with the direction of gravity stabilizes the pose.

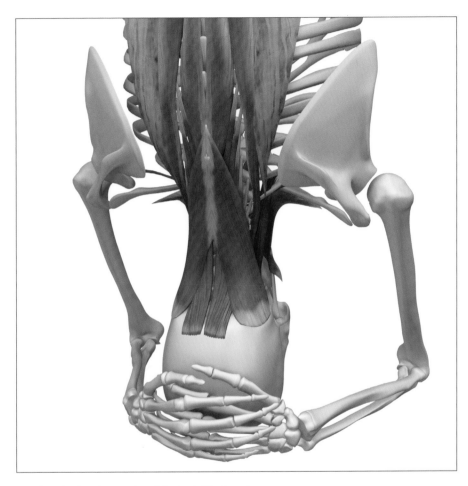

Gently activating the muscles of the back lifts the spine.

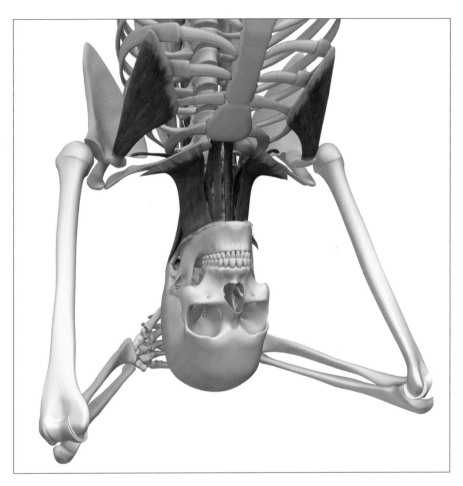

Relaxing the muscles of the front of the neck and activating the pectoralis minor opens the chest and expands the lungs.

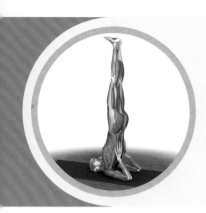

Sarvangasana: Shoulder Stand

The shoulder stand is a restorative inversion. Perform it near the end of your practice to relax.

As an inversion, the shoulder stand has effects that are similar to the headstand. Inverting the body stimulates control mechanisms in the heart and the arteries along the outside of the neck that monitor and adjust blood pressure. Inversions may also positively affect the flow of cerebrospinal fluid in the spinal cord and the brain, flushing regions where the fluid has pooled.

In the shoulder stand, the shoulder joint is extended and the chest opens. Poses like Purvottanasana help one to gain flexibility in moving the shoulders into extension so that the upper arms can be used to open the chest.

Synergizing/Activating

Shoulders and Arms

1. The biceps and brachialis muscles in the arms bend the elbows to press the hands into the back, supporting it and allowing the weight of the body to be shifted away from the neck. Flexor muscles in the forearm shorten to assist this process.

2. The posterior deltoids extend the shoulders away from the trunk and work to press the elbows into the floor.

3. The shoulder blades are drawn away from the neck by the lower trapezius muscle.

4. Two muscles of the rotator cuff, the infraspinatus and teres minor turn the upper arms outward.

Trunk

1. The erector spinae, flowing along the spine, and the rectus abdominis, running from the chest to the pubic bone, lift the trunk.

2. The quadratus lumborum works with the psoas major to support the lower back. Together these neurologically linked muscles wrap around the lumbar spine and stabilize it.

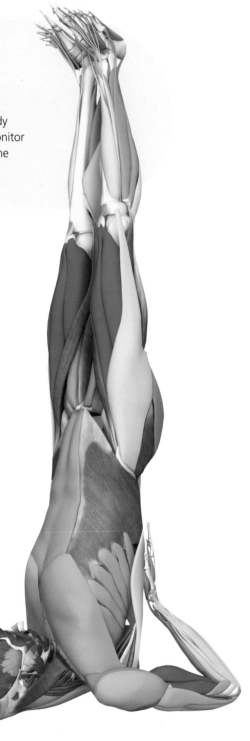

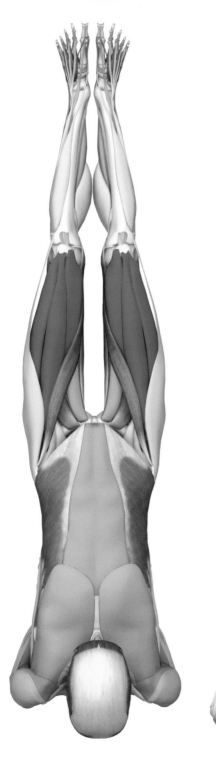

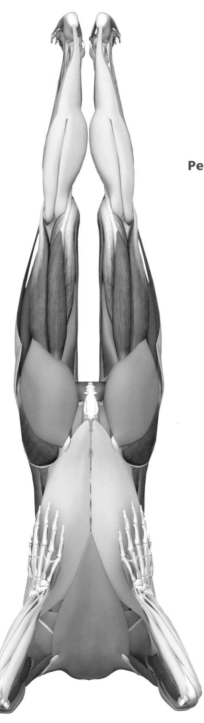

Pelvis and Legs

1. The pelvis is supported and held level by the gluteus maximus in the buttocks and the psoas high at the front of the thighs and in the pelvis.

2. The adductors draw the thighs together.

3. The tensor fascia lata, along the outside of the hip, and the gluteus medius, in the buttocks, turn the hips and thighs inward and counter the outward pull of the buttocks muscle.

4. The quadriceps, along the front of the thighs, straighten the knees.

5. Along the outside of the calf, the peronei turn the feet slightly outward, since there is a tendency for them to tilt inward. This action opens the soles of the feet upward.

6. The feet are drawn toward the head by the tibialis anterior muscles on the front of the shins.

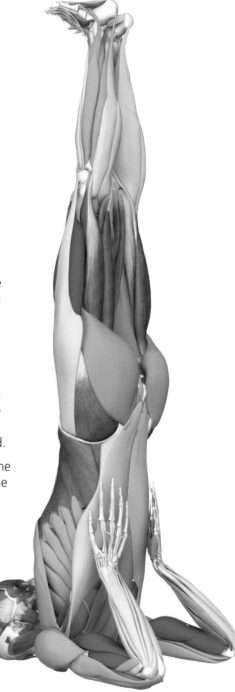

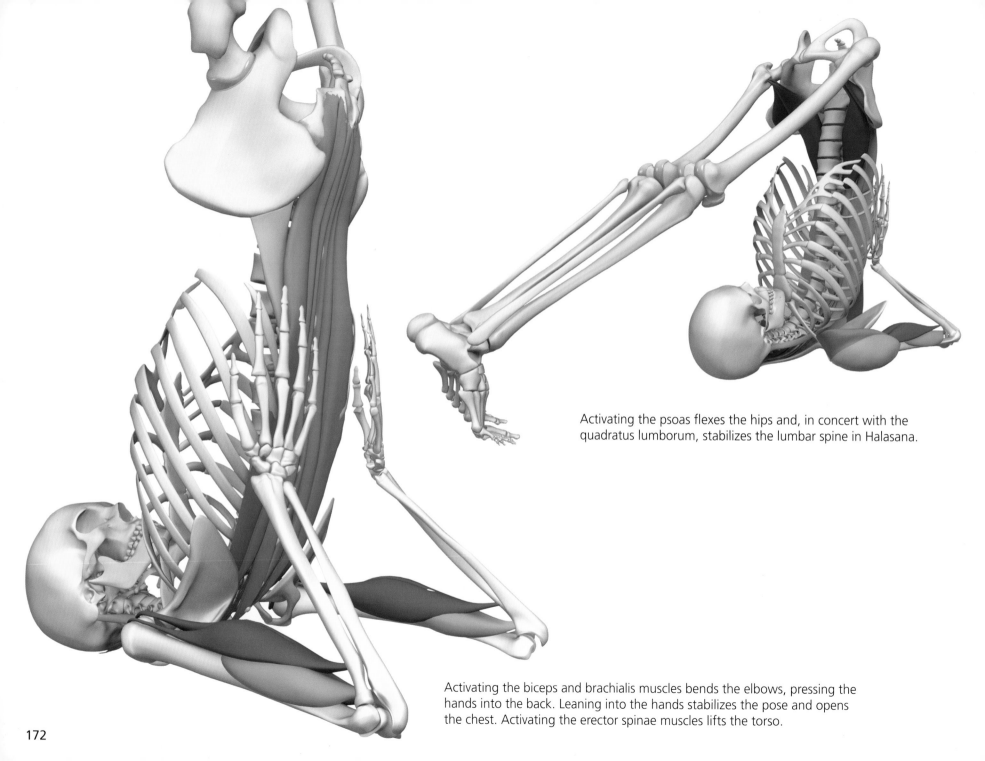

Activating the psoas flexes the hips and, in concert with the quadratus lumborum, stabilizes the lumbar spine in Halasana.

Activating the biceps and brachialis muscles bends the elbows, pressing the hands into the back. Leaning into the hands stabilizes the pose and opens the chest. Activating the erector spinae muscles lifts the torso.

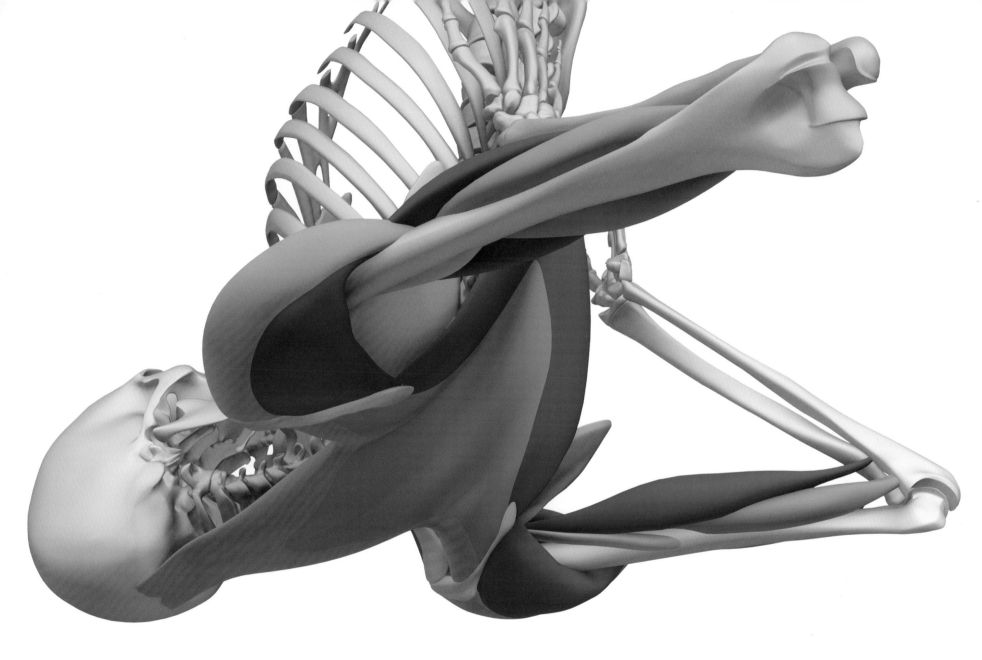

Activating the posterior portion of the deltoids extends the upper arms away from the back. Combining this action with flexing the elbows aids to lift the torso.

Halasana: Plow Pose

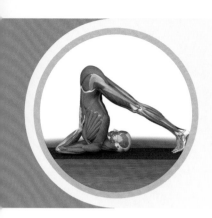

Halasana is one of the restorative poses that is usually performed near the end of the practice. It is also an inversion. Thus, it has beneficial effects on the cardiovascular system and the flow of cerebral spinal fluid.

Synergizing/Activating

1. The biceps flex the elbows. This causes the hands to press into the back, lifting and supporting it while opening the chest.

2. The posterior deltoids extend the humeri toward the floor, further lifting the back.

3. The quadratus lumborum and psoas combine to lift and stabilize the lower back.

4. The psoas and pectineus flex the hips.

5. The adductor longus and brevis draw the thighs toward the midline.

6. The quadriceps extend the knees.

7. The tibialis anterior dorsiflexes the ankles.

8. The peroneus longus and brevis evert the ankles and open the soles of the feet.

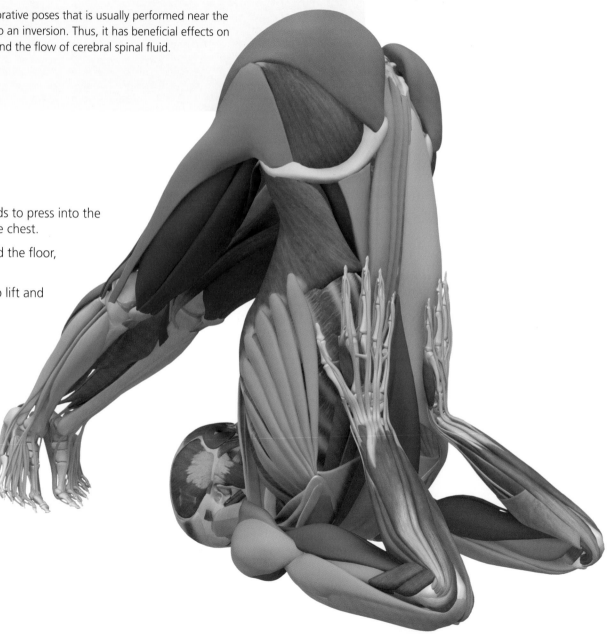

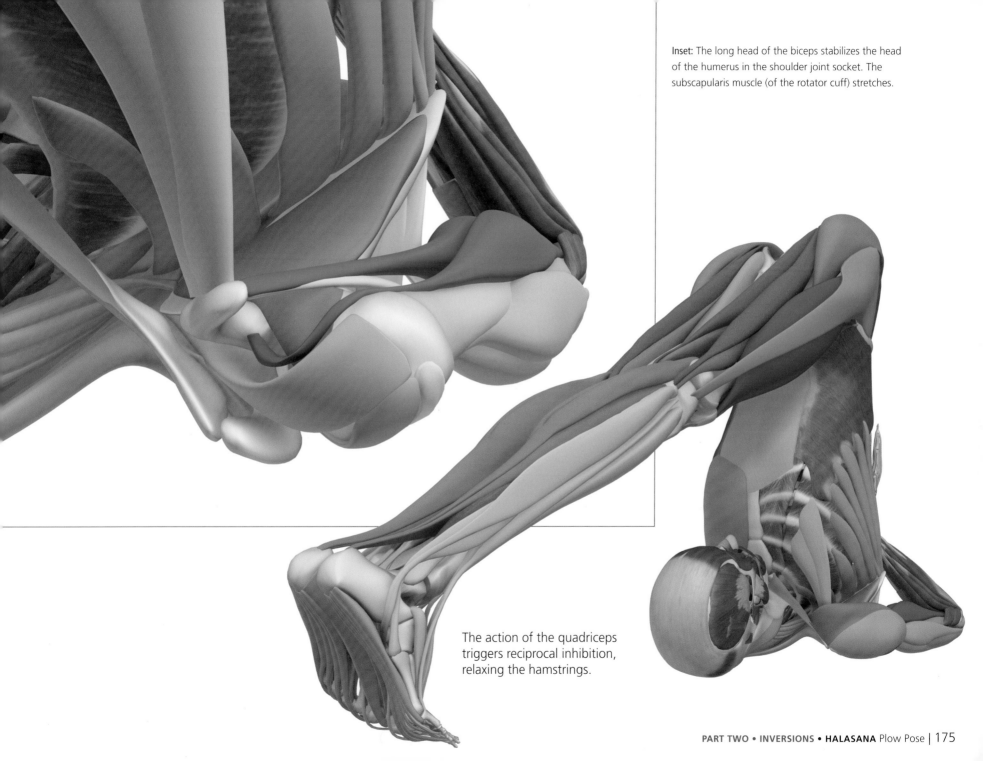

Inset: The long head of the biceps stabilizes the head of the humerus in the shoulder joint socket. The subscapularis muscle (of the rotator cuff) stretches.

The action of the quadriceps triggers reciprocal inhibition, relaxing the hamstrings.

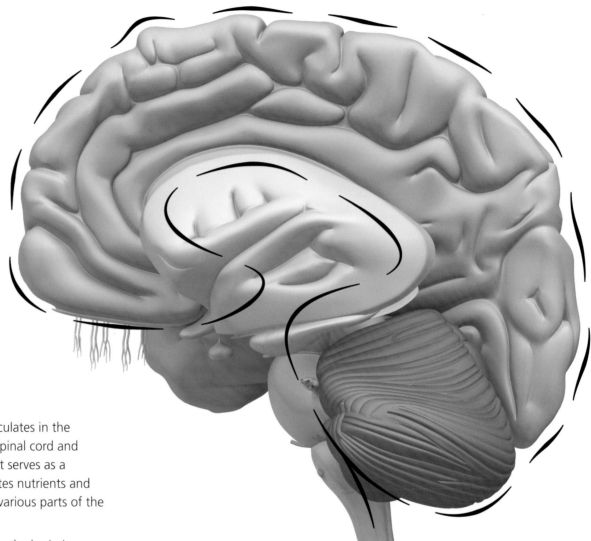

Cerebrospinal Fluid

Cerebrospinal fluid (CSF) is a clear liquid that circulates in the subarachnoid space surrounding the brain and spinal cord and throughout the ventricular system of the brain. It serves as a mechanical cushion against trauma and distributes nutrients and neuroendocrine factors, such as endorphins, to various parts of the central nervous system.

Inverting the body alters the flow of CSF, bathing the brain in endorphins and improving circulation to regions of stagnant flow.

176

Inversions and the Cardiovascular System

Inverting the body affects blood flow, increasing the return of blood from the torso and lower extremities through the inferior vena cava to the heart. The heart pumps more efficiently when the chambers are filled optimally and cardiac output increases. Oxygenated blood is pumped out of the heart through the aorta and distributed to the body.

The aorta and carotid arteries have pressure receptors that aid in regulating blood pressure, maintaining the mean arterial pressure within a narrow range. These receptors respond to increased cardiac output or blood pressure by signaling the brain to increase parasympathetic outflow. This results in a slowing of the heart rate and lowering of the blood pressure. Conversely, when the blood pressure is low (hypotension), signals from the baroreceptors decrease, with cardiac output and blood pressure rising. The net effect is homeostatic balancing of the cardiac output and blood pressure.

Inverting the body in persons with normal blood pressure increases firing of the baroreceptors, thus increasing parasympathetic outflow (from the vagus and glossopharyngeal nerves). The result is a temporarily lowered heart rate and blood pressure.

Always come out of inversions slowly to avoid light-headedness. Child's Pose is excellent for re-equilibrating the body's hemodynamics following inverted poses.

Persons with blood pressure problems, including hypertension or hypotension or glaucoma, should always consult their physician before practicing inversions such as headstand or shoulder stand.

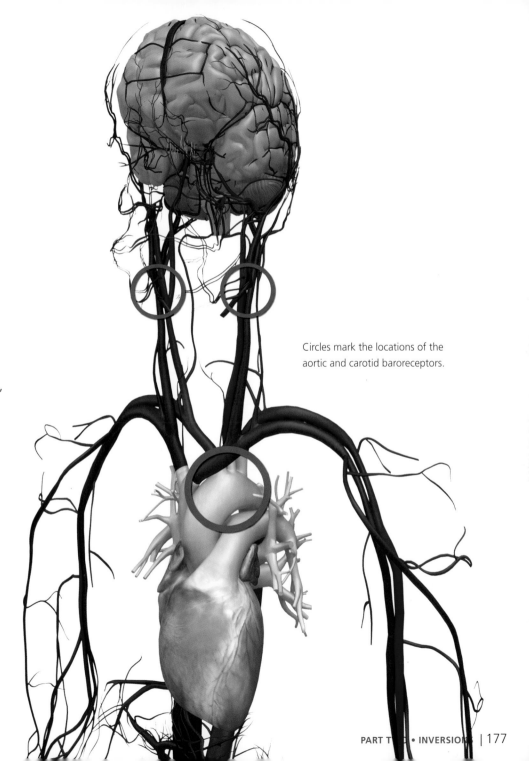

Circles mark the locations of the aortic and carotid baroreceptors.

Restorative Poses

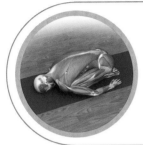

Balasana
Child's Pose
Page 180

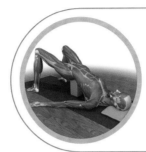

Supported Setu Bandha Sarvangasana
Bridge Pose
Page 182

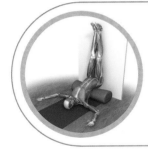

Viparita Karani
Legs-up-the-Wall Pose
Page 184

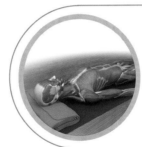

Savasana
Corpse Pose
Page 186

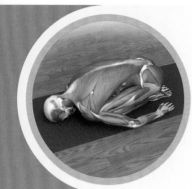

Balasana: Child's Pose

Balasana is a resting pose that can be used any time one feels fatigue during practice. It gently relaxes the muscles on the front of the body while passively stretching the muscles of the back. This action releases the internal organs forward and opens the back of the thorax and lungs.

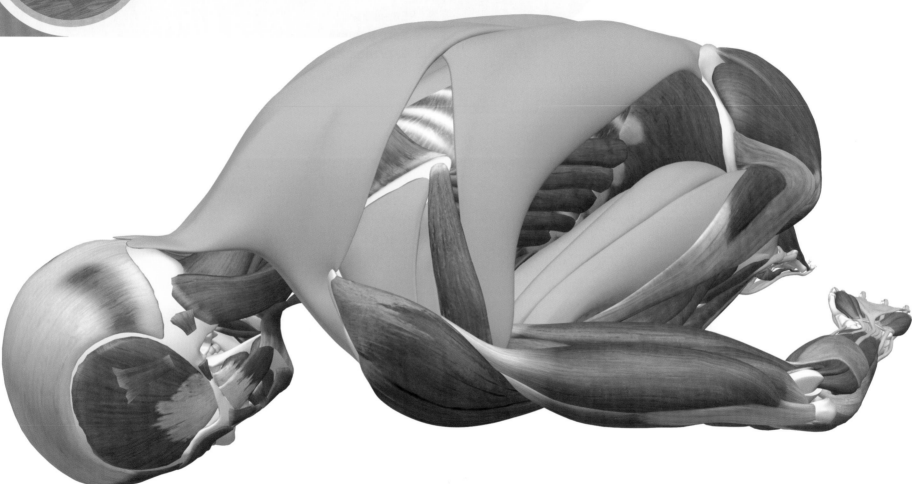

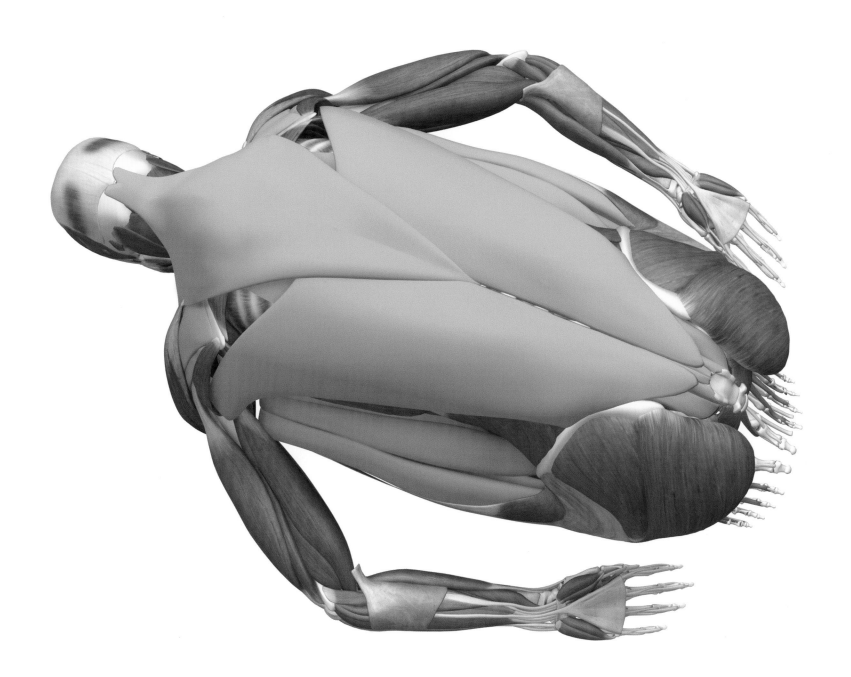

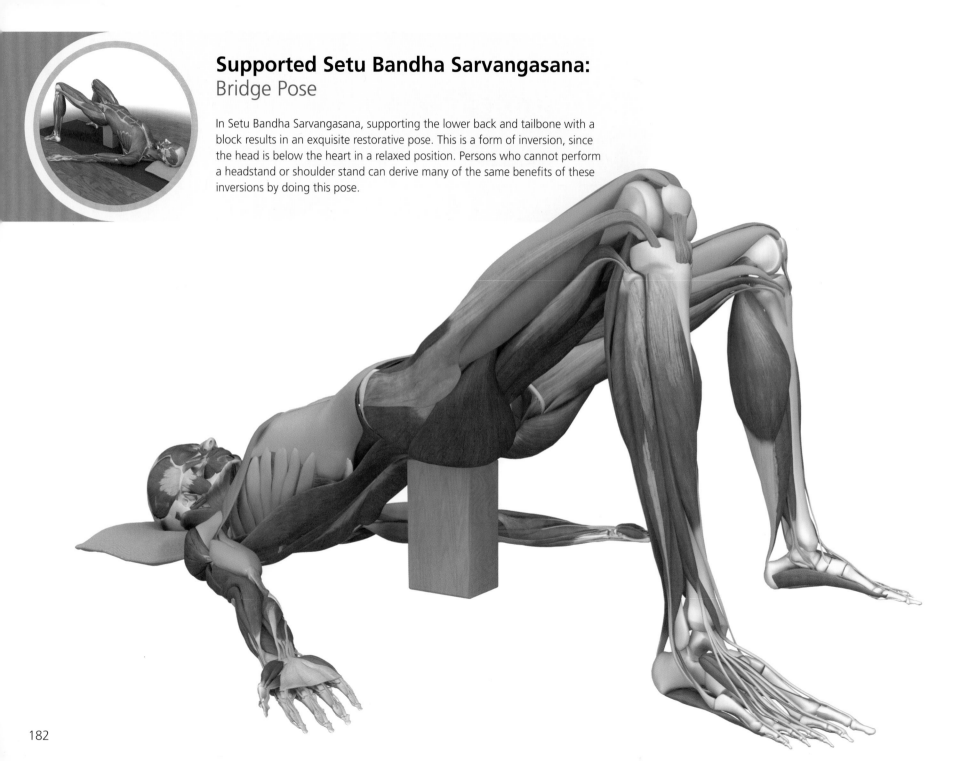

Supported Setu Bandha Sarvangasana:
Bridge Pose

In Setu Bandha Sarvangasana, supporting the lower back and tailbone with a block results in an exquisite restorative pose. This is a form of inversion, since the head is below the heart in a relaxed position. Persons who cannot perform a headstand or shoulder stand can derive many of the same benefits of these inversions by doing this pose.

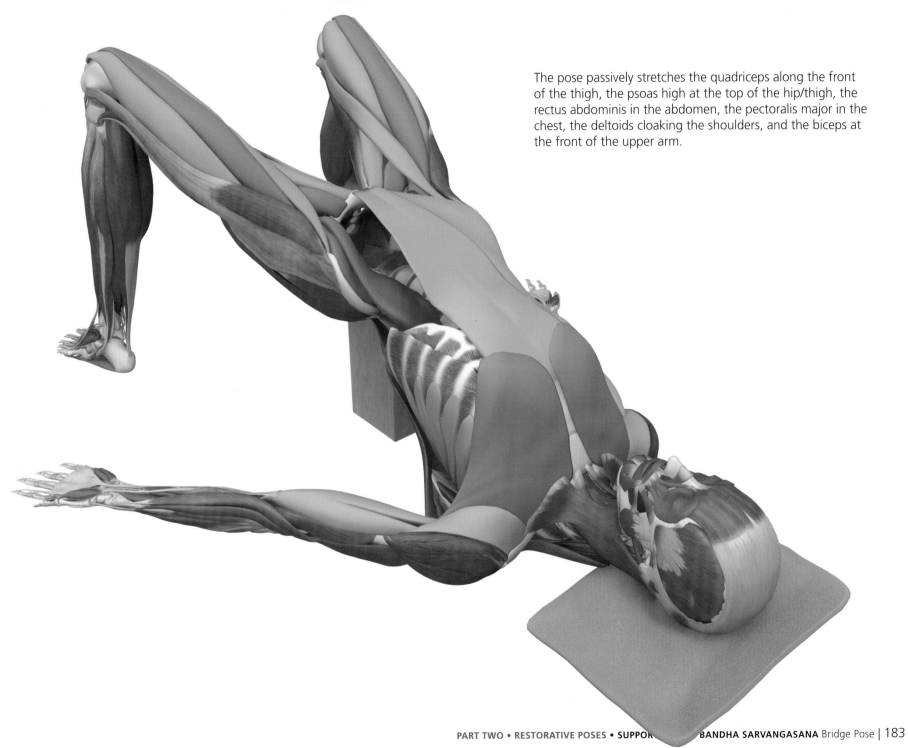

The pose passively stretches the quadriceps along the front of the thigh, the psoas high at the top of the hip/thigh, the rectus abdominis in the abdomen, the pectoralis major in the chest, the deltoids cloaking the shoulders, and the biceps at the front of the upper arm.

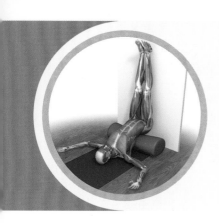

Viparita Karani: Legs-up-the-Wall Pose

In Viparitta Karni, the hips flex and the knees extend to rest the legs against a wall. The pose can also be performed away from the wall, resting the pelvis on a block. The abdomen is passive and resembles a lake. The backs of the legs passively stretch, and the hip flexors relax.

Viparita Karani has cardiovascular effects that are similar to other inversions, including increased return of blood to the heart and activation of the parasympathetic nervous system by the carotid and aortic baroreceptors. As such, it is a useful alternative for practitioners with cervical spine problems who do not wish to practice headstand or shoulder stand.

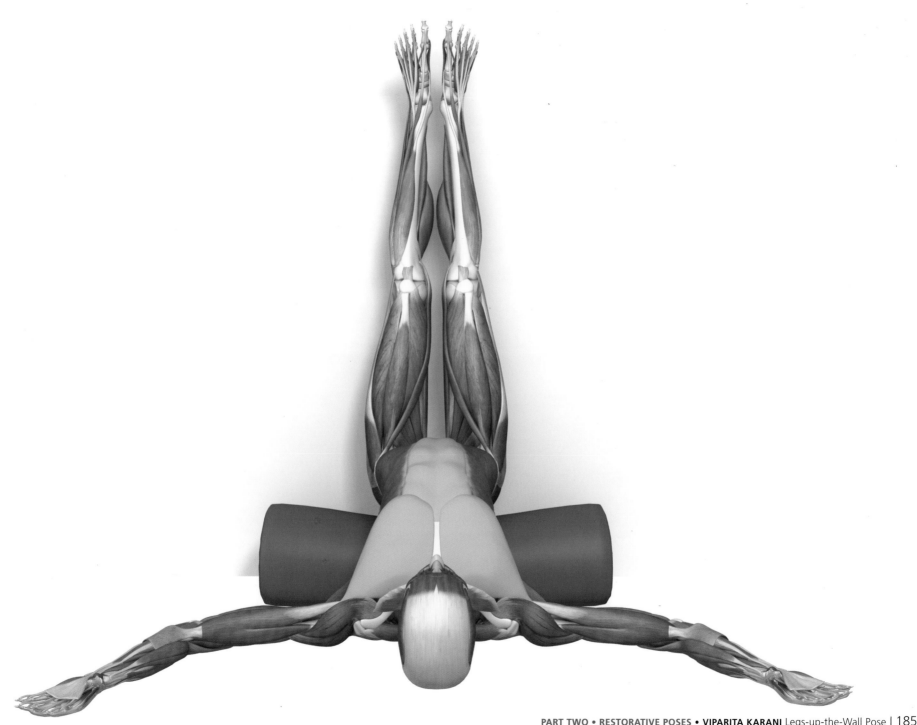

Savasana, or Corpse pose, completes the cycle. The Sun Salutations have reset the muscle lengths in the brain and heated the body. The specific poses have lengthened the muscles surrounding the various joints, stimulating nerve conduction and illuminating the Chakras. The inversions have reconnected us to the parasympathetic nervous system. Now we are ready for deep relaxation.

Theta brain wave patterns predominate in Savasana, with electrical activity oscillating and vibrating at a frequency of 4-8 Hz. This state of brain function engages the intuitive unconscious mind, accessing deep seated memories and connecting to the collective unconscious. Healing occurs in this state. Deeper states of Savasana take the brain wave pattern into Delta (0.5-2 Hz frequency). This is the brain wave state of dreaming.

Passively look inside during Savasana and see the subtle energetic body, illustrated here floating above the physical body.

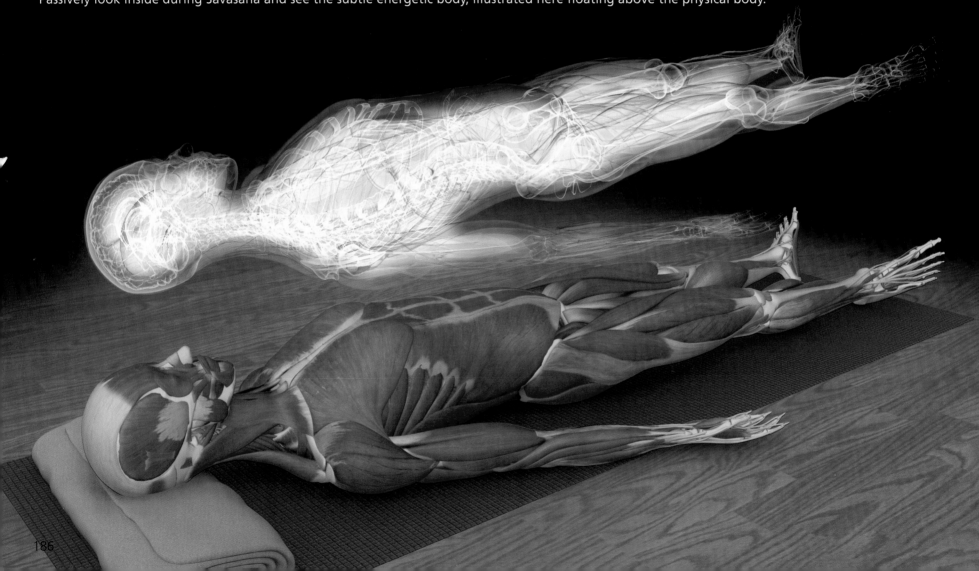

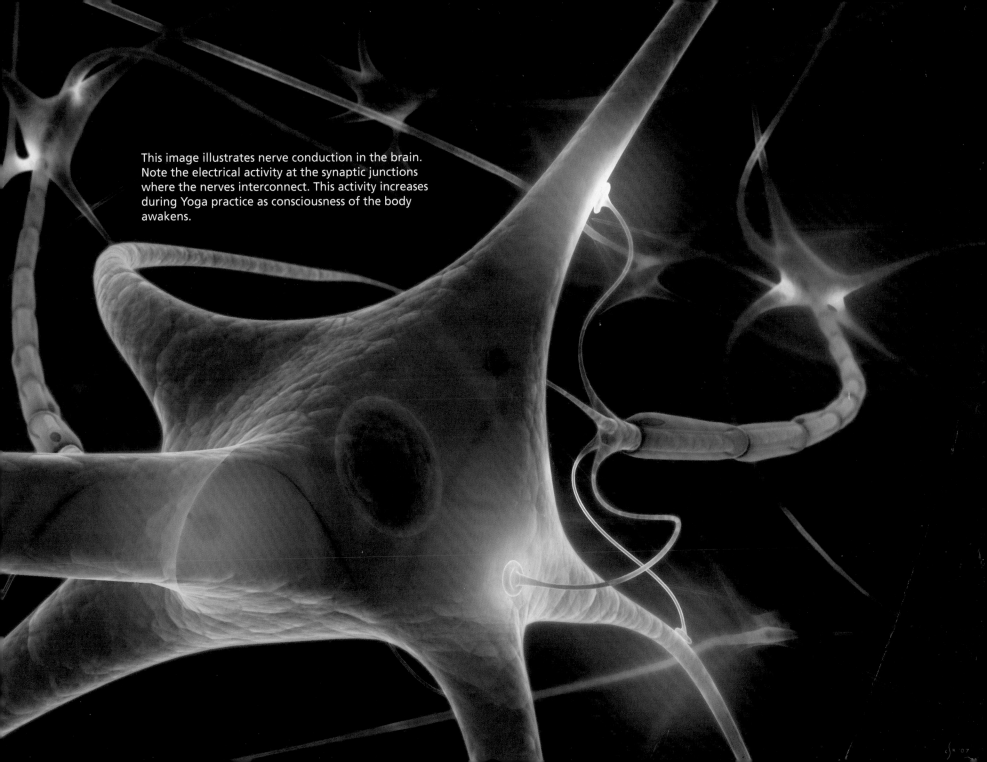

This image illustrates nerve conduction in the brain. Note the electrical activity at the synaptic junctions where the nerves interconnect. This activity increases during Yoga practice as consciousness of the body awakens.

Appendix A:
Guide to Body Movement

Motion of the musculoskeletal system necessarily involves multiple joints, forces applied in many directions, and movement in many planes. A convention exists to describe the basic movements of the musculoskeletal system that can be useful in analyzing the form and function of the Asanas.

The six basic movements of the body take place in three planes:

Coronal plane: Divides the body into front and back. Movements along this plane are called adduction and abduction. Adduction moves the extremity toward the midline, abduction moves the extremity away from the midline.

Sagittal plane: Divides the body into right and left. Movements along this plane are called flexion and extension. Flexion usually moves the extremity forward, except at the knee, where it moves backward. Extension moves the extremity backward.

Transverse plane: Divides the body into upper and lower halves. Movement along this plane is called rotation. Rotation is further classified as medial rotation (toward the midline) or lateral rotation (away from the midline). Medial and lateral rotation are also referred to as internal and external rotation, respectively.

All movements of the body are composed of varying contributions of these six elemental movements.

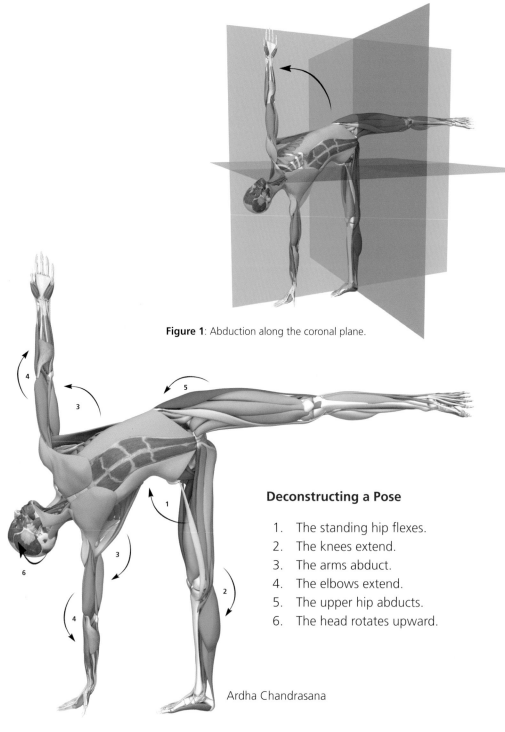

Figure 1: Abduction along the coronal plane.

Deconstructing a Pose

1. The standing hip flexes.
2. The knees extend.
3. The arms abduct.
4. The elbows extend.
5. The upper hip abducts.
6. The head rotates upward.

Ardha Chandrasana

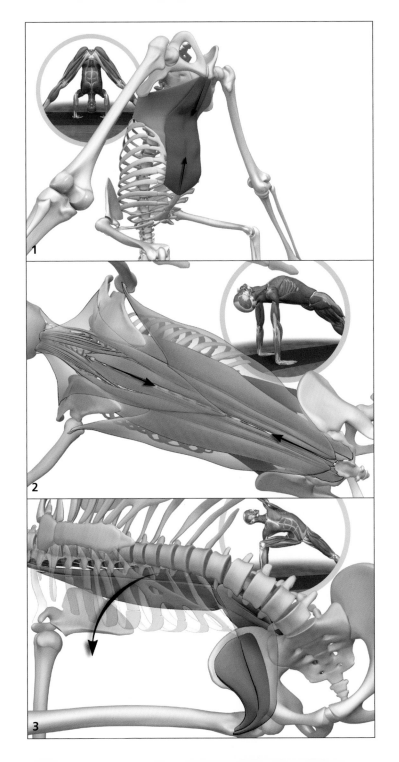

Trunk

Figure 1:
Flexing the Trunk
The abdominal muscles that flex, or bend, the trunk forward include:
- The rectus abdominis: a flat band of muscle extending from the front of the rib cage to the front of the pelvis at the pubis.
- The abdominal obliques: two sheets of muscle with fibers running diagonally from the sides of the rib cage to the iliac bones of the pelvis.
- The transversus abdominis: the innermost sheet of muscle wrapping around the abdomen from the lower ribs to the top of the pelvis.

Figure 2:
Extending the Trunk
The muscles on the back that extend, or arch, the trunk include:
- The quadratus lumborum: a deep rectangular-shaped pair of muscles running alongside the lumbar spine from the top of the back part of the pelvis to the lower ribs and upper lumbar spine.
- The erector spinae muscles: a group of band-like muscles running along the back through its length.
- The latissimus dorsi: a large flat muscle that runs from the back of the pelvis and lower back to the upper arm bone (the humerus).
- The trapezius: a trapezoid-shaped muscle running from the top of the lumbar spine, over the shoulder blades, and up to the back of the neck.

Figure 3:
Laterally Flexing the Trunk
The muscles that bend the trunk to the side include:
- The psoas: a combination of the iliacus and psoas major muscles that run from the the lumbar spine and inside the pelvis to the upper inside part of the thigh bone (the femur).
- The quadratus lumborum: a deep rectangular-shaped muscle running alongside the lumbar spine from the top of the back part of the pelvis to the lower ribs and upper lumbar spine.
- The erector spinae on one side of the back: a group of band-like muscles running along the back through its length.

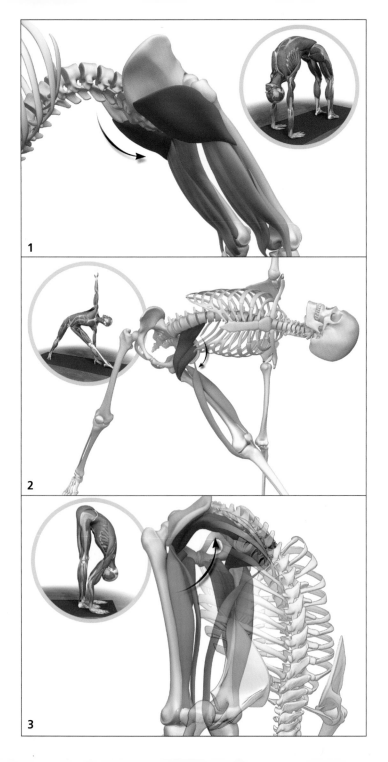

Pelvis

Figure 1:
Tilting the Pelvis Back and Down (Retroversion)
The muscles that tilt the pelvis back and down:
- The gluteus maximus: a large muscle forming the bulk of the buttocks that flows from the back of the pelvis to insert on the side of the thigh bone (femur). Part of this muscle also attaches to the iliotibial band, a sheet-like tendon that attaches to the knee.
- The hamstrings: four tube-shaped muscles running from the back of the pelvis on the sitting bone, the ischial tuberosity, to the top of the lower leg bones (tibia and fibula).

Figure 2:
Tilting the Pelvis Forward (Anteversion)
The muscles that tilt the pelvis forward:
- The psoas: a combination of the iliacus and psoas major muscles that run from the lumbar spine and inside the pelvis to the upper inside part of the thigh bone (the femur).
- The rectus femoris: a long tube-shaped muscle that is part of the quadriceps and runs from the front of the pelvis to the kneecap.
- The sartorius: a narrow band-like muscle that runs diagonally across the surface of the thigh, from the front of the pelvis to the inside of the knee.

Hip

Figure 3:
Flexing the Hip
The muscles that flex the hip upward toward the front of the trunk:
- The psoas: a combination of the iliacus and psoas major muscles that run from the lumbar spine and inside the pelvis to the upper inside part of the thigh bone (the femur).
- The rectus femoris: a long tube-shaped muscle that is part of the quadriceps and that runs from the front of the pelvis to the kneecap.
- The sartorius: a narrow band-like muscle that runs diagonally across the surface of the thigh from the front of the pelvis to the inside of the knee.
- The pectineus: a flat band-like muscle that runs from the front of the pelvis to the inside of the thigh bone.
- The adductor longus and brevis muscles: long, flat, narrow muscles that run from the front of the pelvis to the inside of the femur.

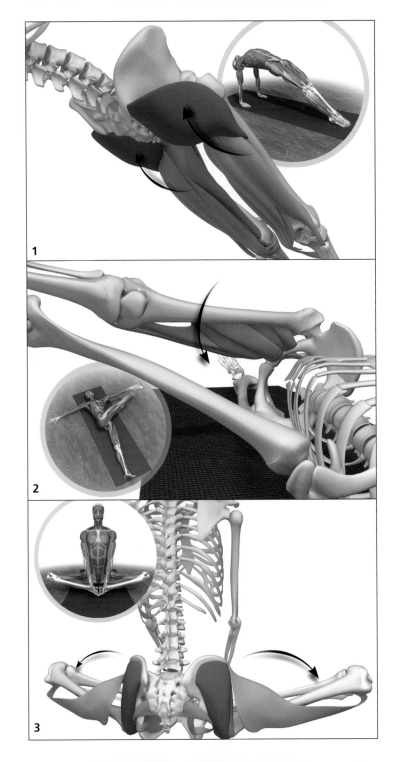

Figure 1:

Extending the Hip

The muscles that extend the hip, opening the front of the pelvis:

- The gluteus maximus: a large muscle forming the bulk of the buttocks that flows from the back of the pelvis to insert on the side of the thigh bone (femur). Part of this muscle also attaches to the iliotibial band, a sheet-like tendon that attaches to the knee.
- The hamstrings: four tube-shaped muscles, three of which run from the back of the pelvis on the sitting bones, and one of which originates from the femur to insert on the top of the lower leg bones (tibia and fibula).

Figure 2:

Drawing the Thigh Toward the Midline (Adduction)

The muscles that adduct the thigh include:

- The adductor group: three muscles running from the front and lower part of the pelvis to the inside of the thigh bone (femur). From the front of the pelvis to the back, these are the adductor longus, adductor brevis, and adductor magnus.
- The pectineus: a flat band-like muscle that runs from the front of the pelvis to the inside of the thigh bone.
- The gracilis: a flat band-like muscle running from the lower front of the pelvis to the inside of the lower leg.

Figure 3:

Drawing the Thigh Away From the Midline (Abduction)

The muscles that abduct the thigh include:

- The gluteus medius and minimus: these muscles form the side part of the buttocks and run from the side of the pelvis to the outside of the thigh bone on the greater trochanter, a large knob-like structure near the top of the femur.
- The tensor fascia lata: a muscle running from the side of the pelvis with a long band-like tendon that inserts onto the front of the main lower leg bone, the tibia.
- The piriformis: a small pyramid-shaped muscle running from the inside of the pelvis to the top outside of the femur, inserting on the inside of the greater trochanter.
- The obturator internus: a narrow tube-like muscle running from the inside of the pelvis to the upper outside of the femur, inserting on the greater trochanter.

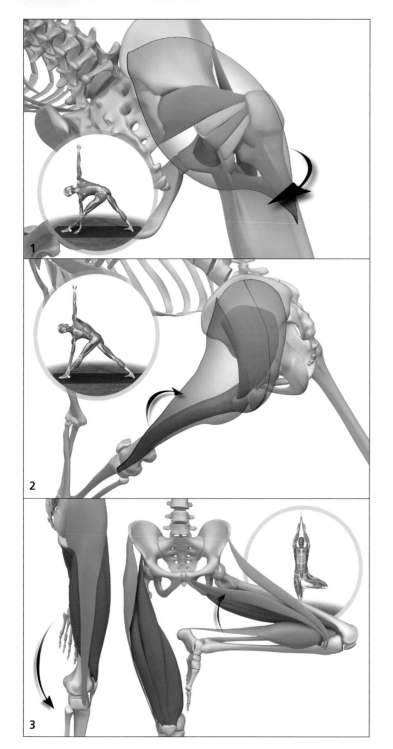

Figure 1:
Turning the Thigh Outward (External Rotation)

The muscles that externally rotate the thigh include:

- The gluteus maximus: a large muscle forming the bulk of the buttocks that flows from the back of the pelvis to insert on the side of the thigh bone (femur). Part of this muscle also attaches to the iliotibial band, a sheet-like tendon that attaches to the knee.
- The adductor magnus: the largest of the adductor muscle group that runs from the lower back of the pelvis, near the sitting bone, to the inside of the femur near the knee.
- The deep external rotators: the piriformis, obturators, gamelli, and quadratus femoris muscles. They run deep to the gluteals and insert on the top part of the femur.
- The sartorius: a narrow, band-like muscle that runs diagonally across the surface of the thigh from the front of the pelvis to the inside of the knee.

Figure 2:
Turning the Thigh Inward (Internal Rotation)

The muscles that internally rotate the thigh include:

- The tensor fascia lata: a muscle running from the side of the pelvis with a long, band-like tendon that inserts onto the front of the main lower leg bone, the tibia.
- The gluteus medius: this muscle forms the side part of the buttocks and runs from the side of the pelvis to the outside of the thigh bone on the greater trochanter, a large knob-like structure near the top of the femur.

Knee

Figure 3 (right leg):
Straightening the Leg (Extension)

The muscles that extend or straighten the knee include:

- The quadriceps: a four-headed muscle on the front of the thigh with three heads running from the femur and one head running from the pelvis to the kneecap (and onto the lower leg).
- The tensor fascia lata: a muscle running from the side of the pelvis with a long band-like tendon that inserts onto the front of the main lower leg bone, the tibia. This muscle assists with the last 30° of extension.

Figure 3 (left leg):
Bending the Leg (Flexion)

The muscles that flex or bend the knee include:

- The hamstrings: four tube-shaped muscles, three of which run from the back of the pelvis on the sitting bones and one of which originates from the femur, to insert on the top of the lower leg bones (tibia and fibula).
- The sartorius: a band-like muscle running diagonally across the thigh, and the gracilis, a muscle running along the inside of the thigh.
- The gastrocnemius: the large muscle forming the calf.

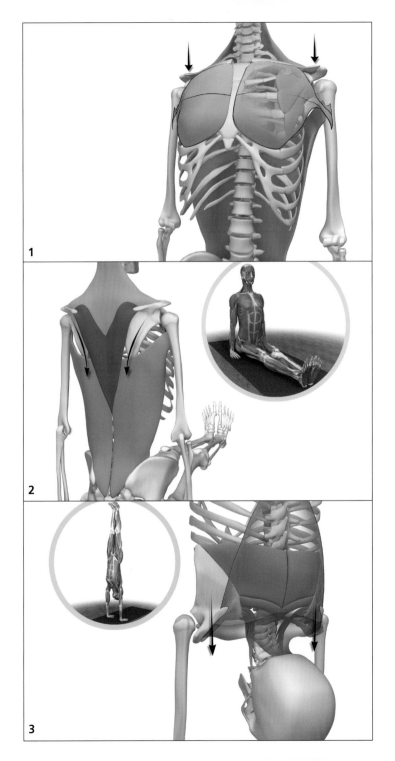

1

2

3

Shoulder Girdle

Figure 1:

Drawing the Shoulders Away From the Neck
(Depressing the Scapulae)

The muscles on the front of the chest that depress the scapulae include:

- The sternal portion of the pectoralis major: this is the lower part of the broad, flat muscle on the front of the chest that runs from the sternum bone at the center of the chest to the upper inside of the humerus.
- The pectoralis minor: a smaller band-like muscle located under the pectoralis major that runs from the upper ribs to the coracoid process, a beak-shaped protrusion of bone on the front of the scapulae.

Figure 2:

The muscles on the back that depress the scapulae include:

- The latissimus dorsi: a large flat muscle that runs from the back of the pelvis and lower back to the upper arm bone (the humerus).
- The lower third of the trapezius: a trapezoid-shaped muscle running from the top of the lumbar spine, over the shoulder blades, and up to the back of the neck.

Figure 3:

Lifting or Elevating the Shoulder Girdle

The muscles that elevate the shoulder girdle include:

- The upper third of the trapezius: a trapezoid-shaped muscle running from the top of the lumbar spine, over the shoulder blades, and up to the back of the neck.
- The levator scapulae: a group of small tube-like muscles running from the top of the shoulder blades to the sides of the upper four vertebrae in the neck.
- The rhomboids: two flat muscles, the rhomboid major and minor, that run from the inner border of the shoulder blades to the midline of the back at the spine.

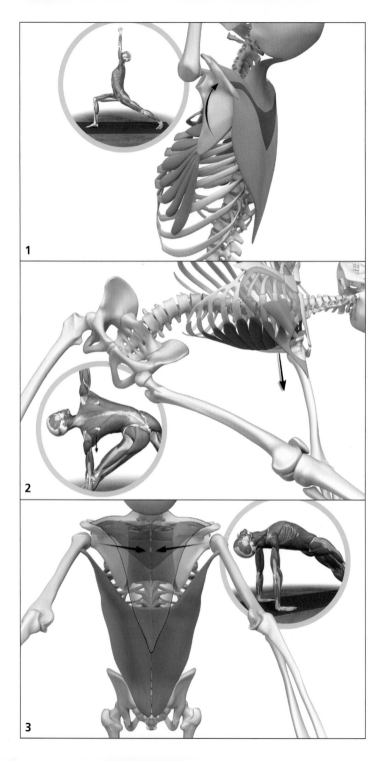

Figure 1:

Rotating the Shoulder Blade Upward

The muscles that rotate the scapulae upward include:

- The serratus anterior: a group of narrow, flat muscles that run from the inner surface of the medial border of the scapula to the front part of the rib cage.
- The upper and middle thirds of the trapezius: a trapezoid-shaped muscle running from the top of the lumbar spine, over the shoulder blades, and up to the back of the neck.

Figure 2:

Moving the Shoulder Blades Away From the Midline (Protraction or Abduction)

The muscles that protract the shoulder blades include:

- The serratus anterior: the group of narrow flat muscles that run from the inner surface of the medial border of the scapula to the front part of the rib cage.
- The pectoralis major: the broad flat muscle on the front of the chest that runs from the sternum bone at the center of the chest and from the collar bone to the upper inside of the humerus.
- The pectoralis minor: a smaller band-like muscle located under the pectoralis major that runs from the upper ribs to the coracoid process, a beak-shaped protrusion of bone on the front of the scapula.

Figure 3:

Drawing the Shoulder Blades Toward the Midline of the Back (Retraction)

The muscles that retract the shoulder blades toward the midline include:

- The rhomboids: two flat muscles, the rhomboid major and minor, that run from the inner border of the shoulder blades to the midline of the back at the spine.
- The middle third of the trapezius: a trapezoid-shaped muscle running from the top of the lumbar spine, over the shoulder blades, and up to the back of the neck.
- The latissimus dorsi: the large flat muscle that runs from the back of the pelvis and lower back to the upper arm bone (the humerus).

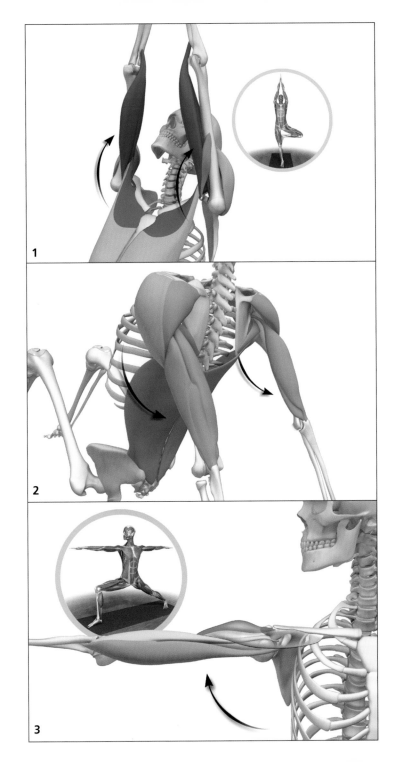

Shoulder and Upper Arms

Figure 1:

Raising the Arms Above the Head (Flexion)

The muscles that flex the arms include:

- The anterior portion of the deltoids: the large muscle that covers the shoulders and runs from the top of the shoulder blade and clavicle to the outside of the humerus.
- The biceps: the large muscle on the front of the upper arms.
- The coracobrachialis: the thin tube-like muscle running from the coracoid process to the mid-portion of the humerus.
- The pectoralis major (sternoclavicular or upper portion): the broad flat muscle on the front of the chest that runs from the sternum bone at the center of the chest and from the collar bone to the upper inside of the humerus.

Figure 2:

Moving the Arms Backward (Extension)

The muscles that extend the arms include:

- The triceps (long head): the large muscle on the back of the upper arms has three heads. The long head originates from the lower border of the shoulder socket, inserting on the olecranon process of the ulna (forearm bone).
- The latissimus dorsi: a large flat muscle that runs from the back of the pelvis and lower back to the upper arm bone (the humerus).
- The posterior third of the deltoid: the large muscle that covers the shoulders and runs from the top of the shoulder blade and clavicle to the outside of the humerus.

Figure 3:

Moving the Arm From the Midline (Abduction)

The muscles that abduct the arms include:

- The lateral portion of the deltoids. The large muscle that covers the shoulders and runs from the top of the shoulder blade and clavicle to the outside of the humerus is divided into thirds. These are the front (anterior), side (lateral), and back (posterior) portions of the muscle.
- The long head of the biceps. The large muscle on the front of the upper arms has a long and a short head. The long head originates from the top of the shoulder socket (glenoid), and the short head originates from the beak-like coracoid process at the front of the scapula. Both heads combine to insert onto the radius bone of the forearm.
- The supraspinatus. The muscle running from a depression on the back of the shoulder blade above the spine of the scapula to the head of the humerus initiates abduction of the upper arm.

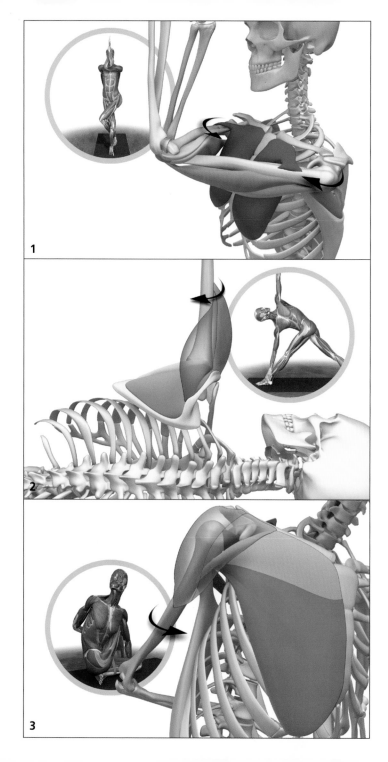

Figure 1:

Moving the Arms Toward the Midline of the Body (Adduction)

The muscles that adduct the arms include:

- The pectoralis major: the broad flat muscle on the front of the chest that runs from the sternum bone at the center of the chest and from the collar bone to the upper inside of the humerus.
- The teres major: the narrow band-like muscle running from the lower border of the scapula to the humerus.
- The latissimus dorsi: the large flat muscle that runs from the back of the pelvis and lower back to the upper arm bone (the humerus).
- The long head of the triceps: the large muscle on the back of the upper arms has three heads. The long head originates from the lower border of the shoulder socket, and the medial and lateral heads originate from the humerus, inserting onto the ulna bone of the forearm.

Figure 2:

Turning the Arm Outward (External Rotation)

The muscles that externally rotate the upper arm (humerus) include:

- The posterior third of the deltoid. The large muscle that covers the shoulders and runs from the top of the shoulder blade and clavicle to the outside of the humerus is divided into thirds. These are the front (anterior), side (lateral), and back (posterior) portions of the muscle.
- The infraspinatus: the muscle running from a depression on the back of the shoulder blade below the spine of the scapula to the head of the humerus.
- The teres minor: the small, narrow muscle originating from the lower outside border of the scapula and running to the head of the humerus, inserting just behind the infraspinatus.

Figure 3:

Turning the Arm Inward (Internal Rotation)

The muscles that internally rotate the upper arm include:

- The sternocostal portion of the pectoralis major. This is the lower part of the broad, flat muscle on the front of the chest that runs from the sternum bone at the center of the chest to the upper inside of the humerus.
- The front or anterior portion of the deltoids. The large muscle that covers the shoulders and runs from the top of the shoulder blade and clavicle to the outside of the humerus is divided into thirds. These are the front (anterior), side (lateral), and back (posterior) portions of the muscle.
- The subscapularis: the fan-shaped flat muscle originating from the front surface of the scapula and running in front of the shoulder joint to attach to a small knob on the humeral head, the lesser tuberosity.
- The latissimus dorsi: the large flat muscle that runs from the back of the pelvis and lower back to the upper arm bone (the humerus).
- The teres major: the narrow band-like muscle running from the lower border of the scapula to the humerus.

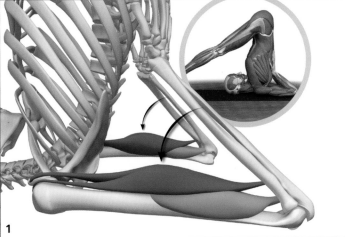

1

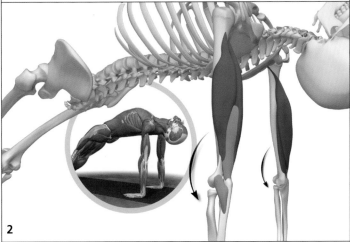

2

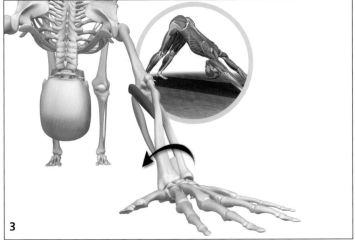

3

Elbow

Figure 1:

Bending (Flexing) the Elbow

The muscles that flex the elbow include:

- The biceps brachii: the large muscle on the front of the upper arms has a long and short head. The long head originates from the top of the shoulder socket (glenoid). The short head originates from the beak-like coracoid process at the front of the scapula. Both heads combine to insert onto the radius bone of the forearm.
- The brachialis: the muscle located under the biceps just above the elbow on the front of the humerus, originating from the humerus and inserting on the ulna bone of the forearm.

Figure 2:

Straightening (Extending) the Elbow

The muscles that extend the elbow include:

- The triceps. This large muscle on the back of the upper arms has three heads. The long head originates from the lower border of the shoulder socket, and the medial and lateral heads originate from the humerus, inserting onto the ulna bone of the forearm.
- The anconeus: the small muscle on the outside of the elbow, running from the back part of the lateral condyle of the elbow to the ulna bone of the forearm.

Forearm

Figure 3:

Turning the Palm to Face Downward (Pronating the Forearm)

The muscles that pronate the forearm include:

- The pronator teres: the flat band-like muscle originating at the humerus on the inside of the elbow and crossing over to insert onto the shaft of the radius bone of the forearm.
- The pronator quadratus: this flat square-shaped muscle in the forearm bridges the forearm bones, the radius and ulna.

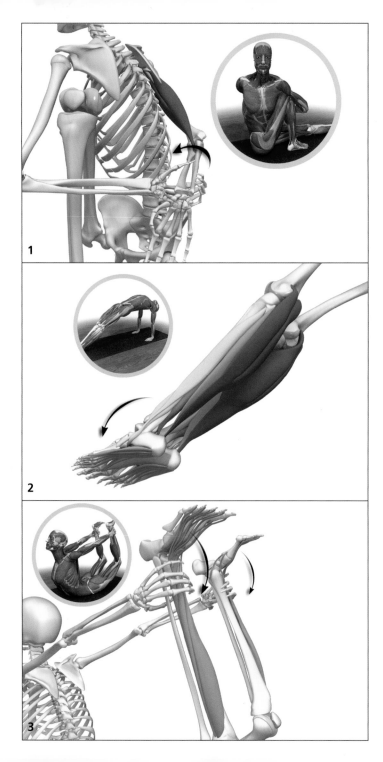

Figure 1:

Turning the Palm Upward (Supinating the Forearm)

The muscles that supinate the forearm include:

1. The biceps brachii. The large muscle on the front of the upper arms has a long and short head. The long head originates from the top of the shoulder socket (glenoid). The short head originates from the beak-like coracoid process at the front of the scapula. Both heads combine to insert onto the radius bone of the forearm.
2. The supinator: the thin sheet-like muscle originating from the outer surface of the humerus at the elbow and ulna, then wrapping around to insert on the radius bone of the forearm.

Ankle

Figure 2:

Pressing the Sole of the Foot Downward (Plantar Flexion)

The muscles that plantar flex the foot include:

1. The gastrocnemius: the large two-headed muscle originating from the back of the femur and inserting onto the heel bone (calcaneus) via the Achilles tendon.
2. The soleus: the bulky muscle under the gastrocnemius that originates from the tibia and inserts onto the heel bone via the Achilles tendon.
3. The peroneus longus and brevis: long, thin tube-like muscles originating from the side of the fibula and inserting on the bottom and outside of the foot, respectively.
4. The tibialis posterior: the deep muscle originating from the back of the shin bone (tibia) and wrapping around the inside of the ankle to insert on the bottom of the foot.
5. The flexor hallucis longus: the deep muscle originating from the back of the fibula and wrapping around the inside of the ankle to insert on the bottom of the big toe.

Figure 3:

Drawing the Foot Toward the Shin (Dorsiflexion)

The muscles that dorsiflex the foot include:

1. The tibialis anterior: the long flat muscle originating from the front of the shin bone (tibia) and inserting on the inner surface of the foot.
2. The extensor hallucis longus: the smaller tube-like muscle underneath the tibialis anterior that originates from the fibula and inserts on the top of the big toe.
3. The extonsor digitorum longus: the long thin muscle originating from the outside of the shin and inserting onto the tops of the toes.

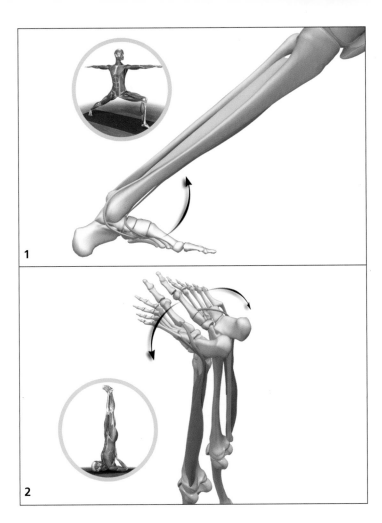

Figure 1:

Tilting the Foot Inward (Inversion)

The muscles that invert the foot include:

1. The tibialis anterior: the long flat muscle originating from the front of the shin bone (tibia) and inserting on the inner surface of the foot.
2. The tibialis posterior: the deep muscle originating from the back of the shin bone (tibia) and wrapping around the inside of the ankle to insert on the bottom of the foot.

Figure 2:

Tilting the Foot Outward (Eversion)

The muscles that evert the foot include:

1. The peroneus longus and brevis: long thin tube-like muscles originating from the side of the fibula and inserting on the bottom and outside of the foot, respectively.

Appendix B:
Index of Anatomy

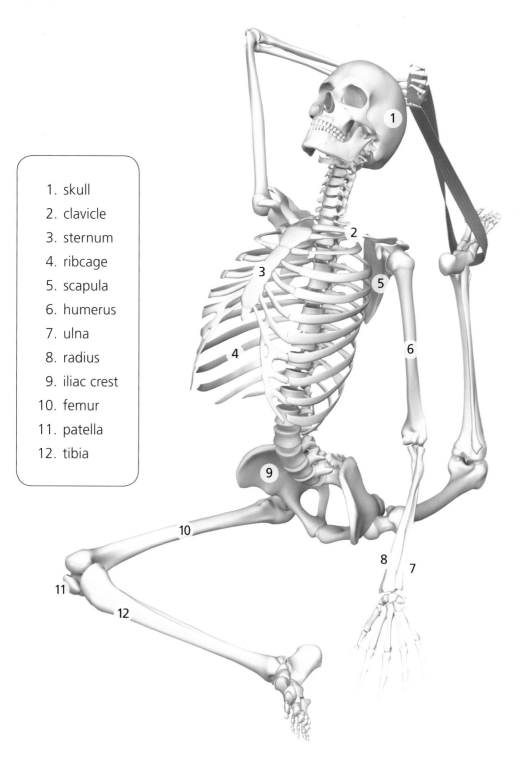

1. skull
2. clavicle
3. sternum
4. ribcage
5. scapula
6. humerus
7. ulna
8. radius
9. iliac crest
10. femur
11. patella
12. tibia

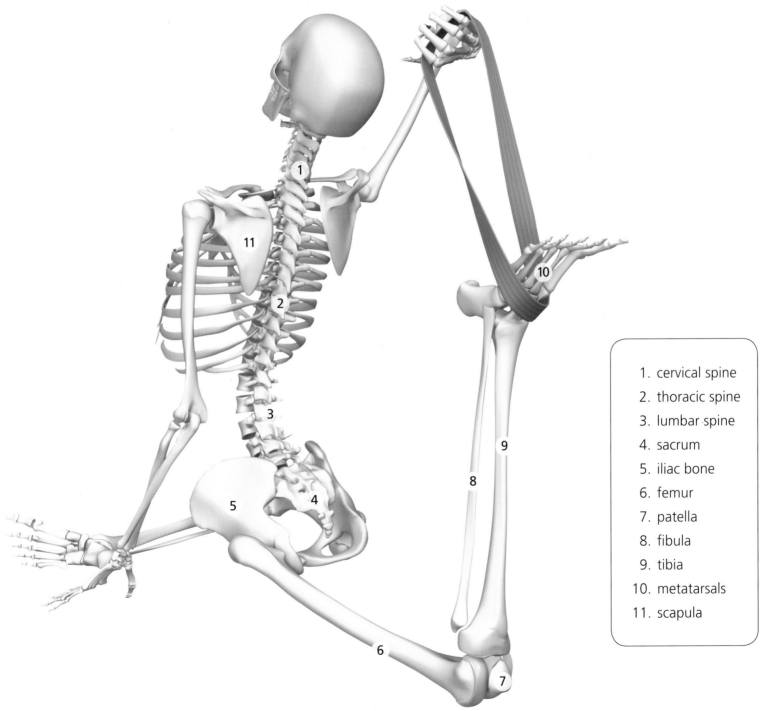

1. cervical spine
2. thoracic spine
3. lumbar spine
4. sacrum
5. iliac bone
6. femur
7. patella
8. fibula
9. tibia
10. metatarsals
11. scapula

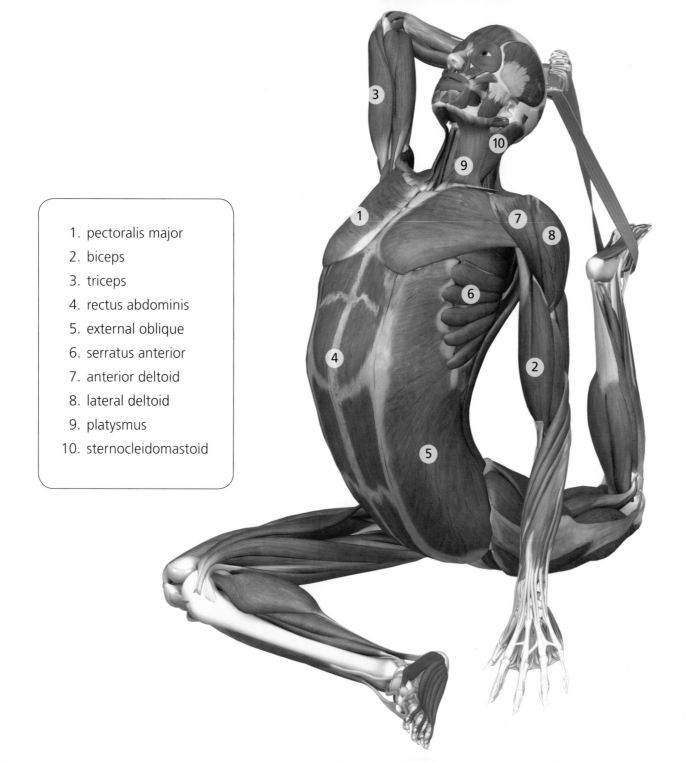

1. pectoralis major
2. biceps
3. triceps
4. rectus abdominis
5. external oblique
6. serratus anterior
7. anterior deltoid
8. lateral deltoid
9. platysmus
10. sternocleidomastoid

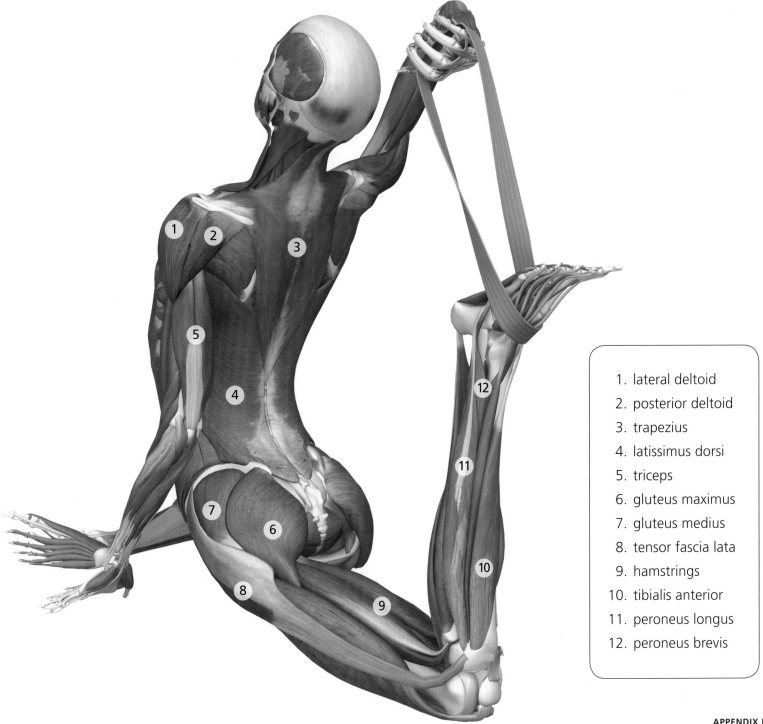

1. lateral deltoid
2. posterior deltoid
3. trapezius
4. latissimus dorsi
5. triceps
6. gluteus maximus
7. gluteus medius
8. tensor fascia lata
9. hamstrings
10. tibialis anterior
11. peroneus longus
12. peroneus brevis

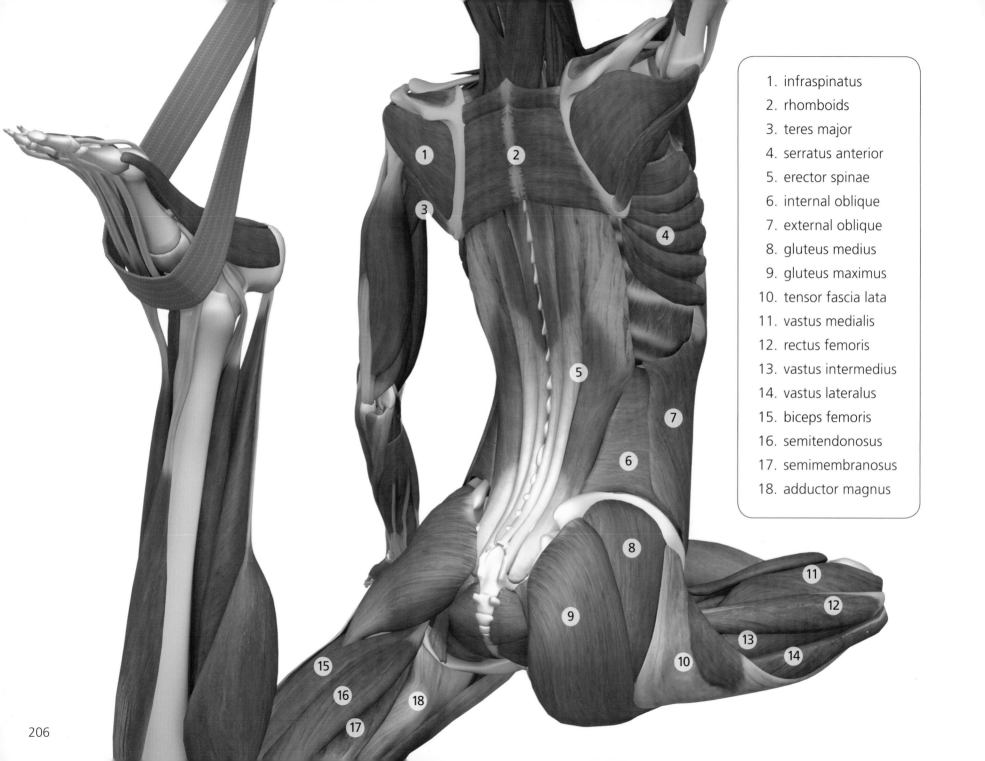

1. infraspinatus
2. rhomboids
3. teres major
4. serratus anterior
5. erector spinae
6. internal oblique
7. external oblique
8. gluteus medius
9. gluteus maximus
10. tensor fascia lata
11. vastus medialis
12. rectus femoris
13. vastus intermedius
14. vastus lateralus
15. biceps femoris
16. semitendonosus
17. semimembranosus
18. adductor magnus

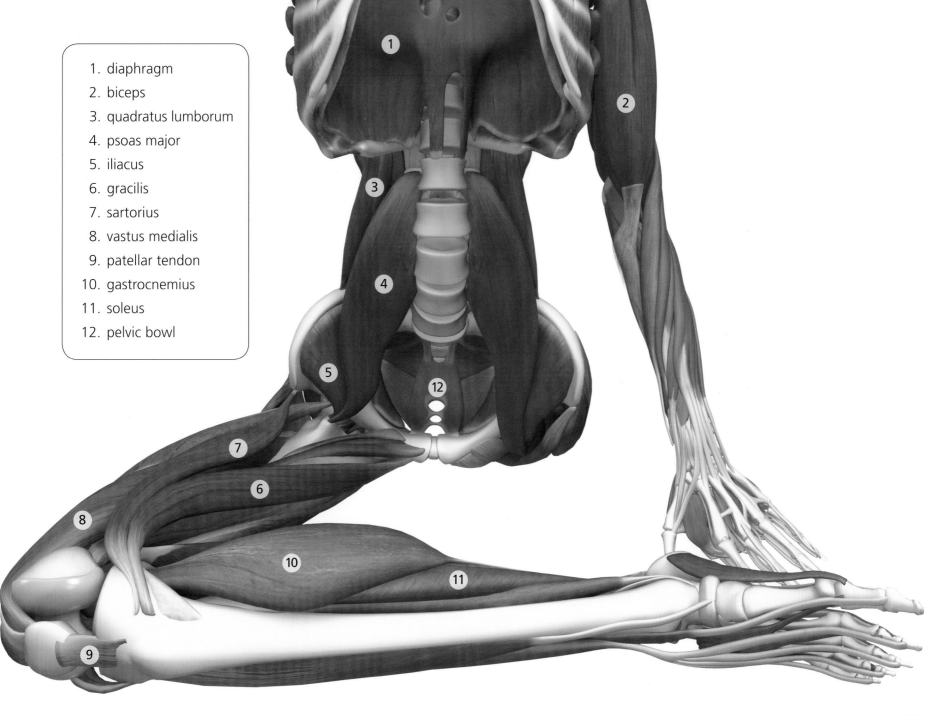

1. diaphragm
2. biceps
3. quadratus lumborum
4. psoas major
5. iliacus
6. gracilis
7. sartorius
8. vastus medialis
9. patellar tendon
10. gastrocnemius
11. soleus
12. pelvic bowl

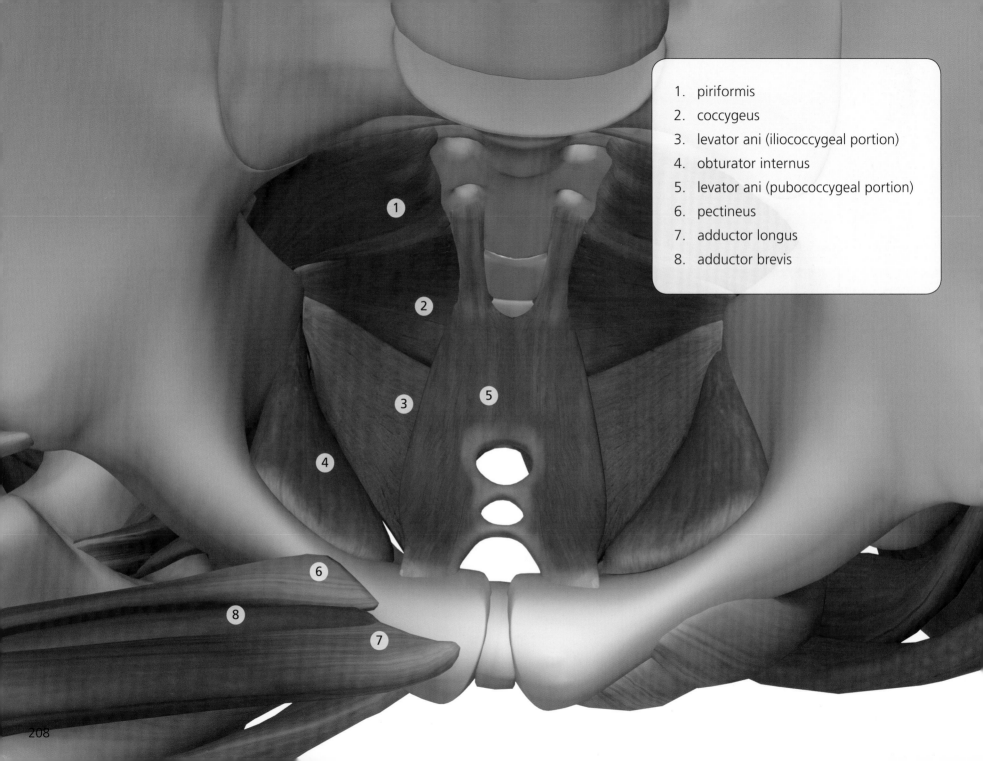

1. piriformis
2. coccygeus
3. levator ani (iliococcygeal portion)
4. obturator internus
5. levator ani (pubococcygeal portion)
6. pectineus
7. adductor longus
8. adductor brevis

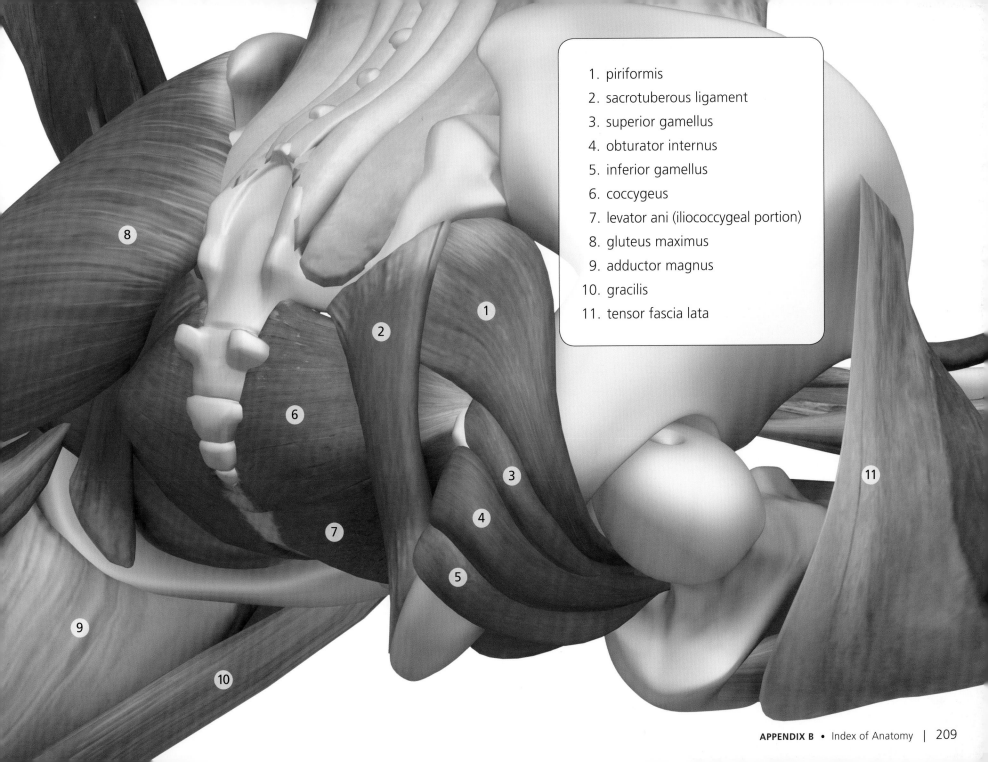

1. piriformis
2. sacrotuberous ligament
3. superior gamellus
4. obturator internus
5. inferior gamellus
6. coccygeus
7. levator ani (iliococcygeal portion)
8. gluteus maximus
9. adductor magnus
10. gracilis
11. tensor fascia lata

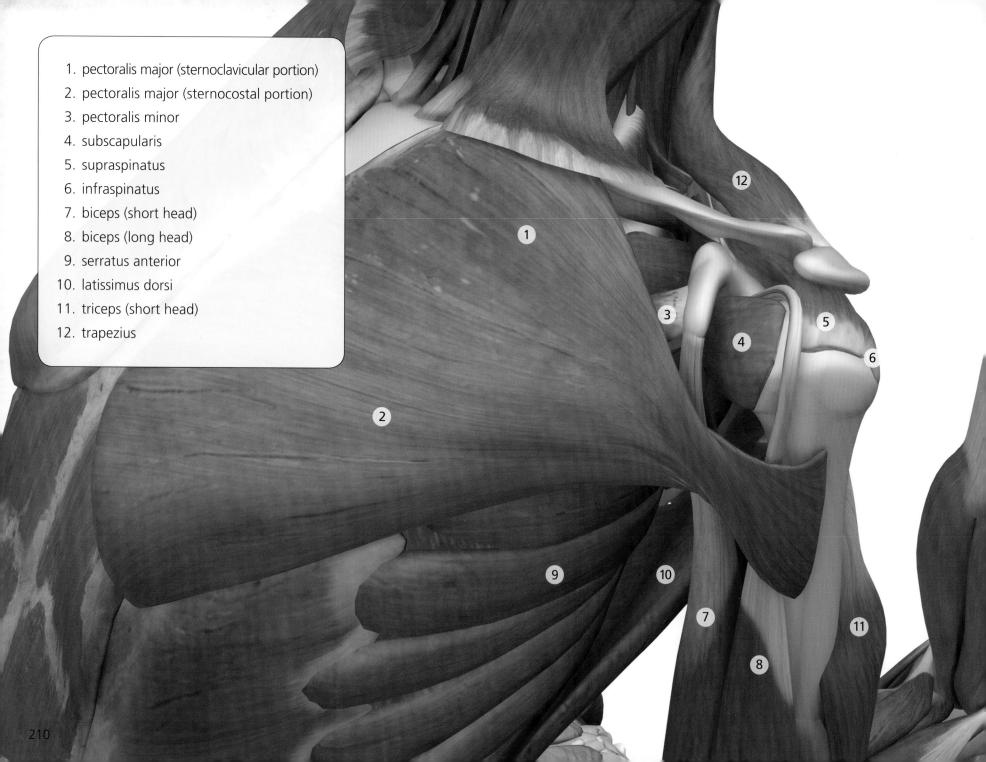

1. pectoralis major (sternoclavicular portion)
2. pectoralis major (sternocostal portion)
3. pectoralis minor
4. subscapularis
5. supraspinatus
6. infraspinatus
7. biceps (short head)
8. biceps (long head)
9. serratus anterior
10. latissimus dorsi
11. triceps (short head)
12. trapezius

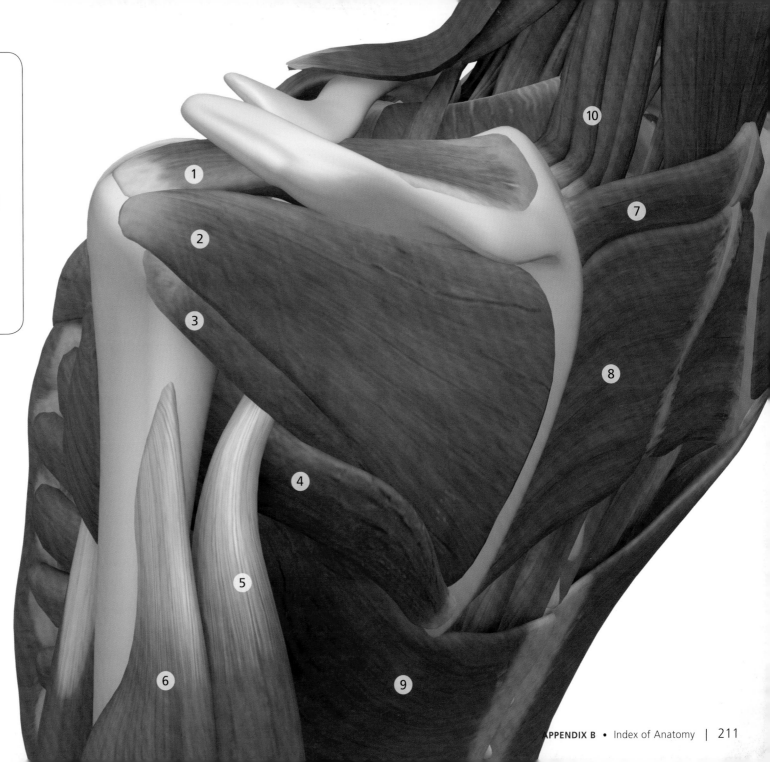

1. supraspinatus
2. infraspinatus
3. teres minor
4. teres major
5. triceps (long head)
6. triceps (short head)
7. rhomboid minor
8. rhomboid major
9. latissimus dorsi
10. levator scapulae

Appendix C:
Index of Poses

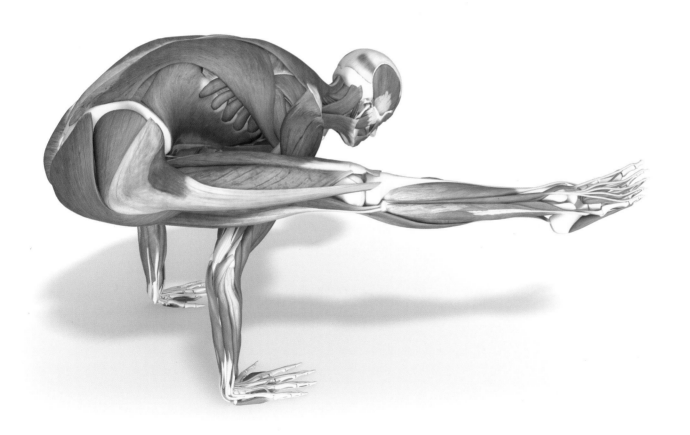